Germ Line Mutations Associated Leukemia

Edited by Zhan He Wu

Published in London, United Kingdom

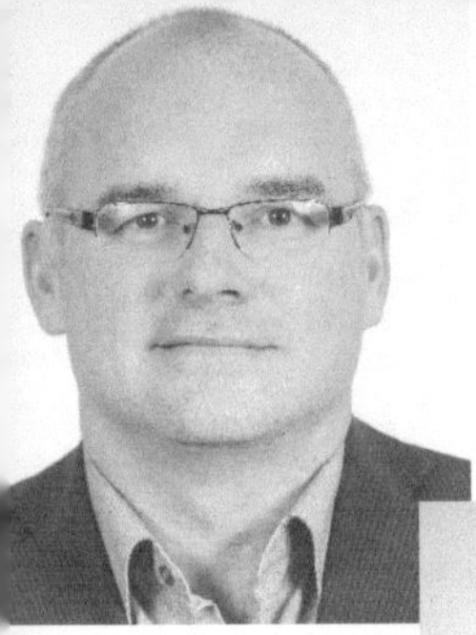
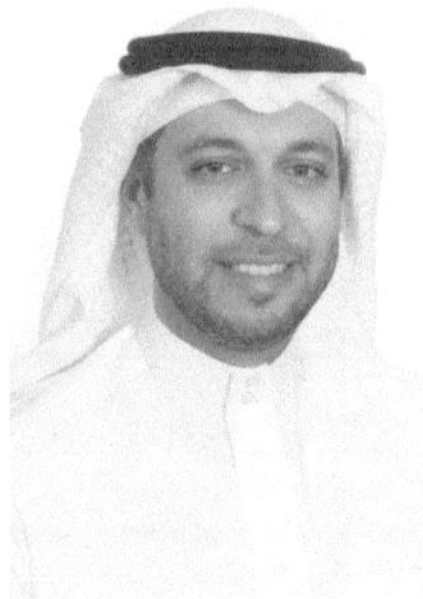
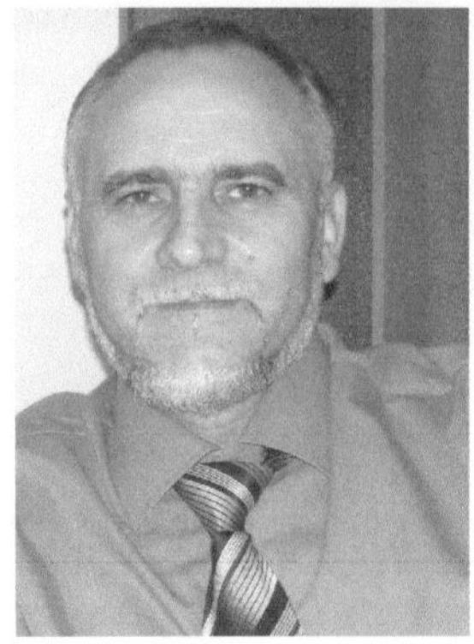
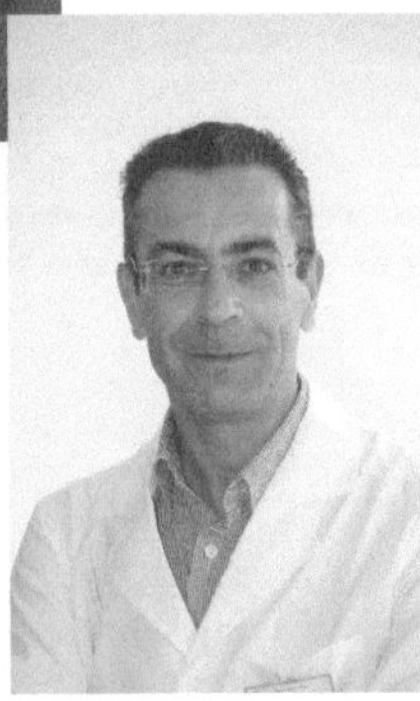
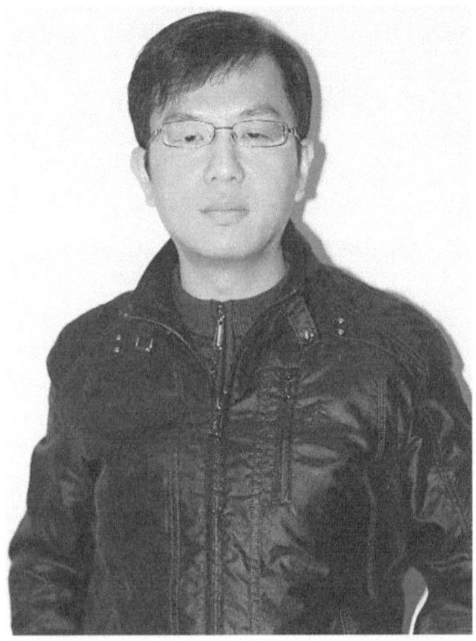
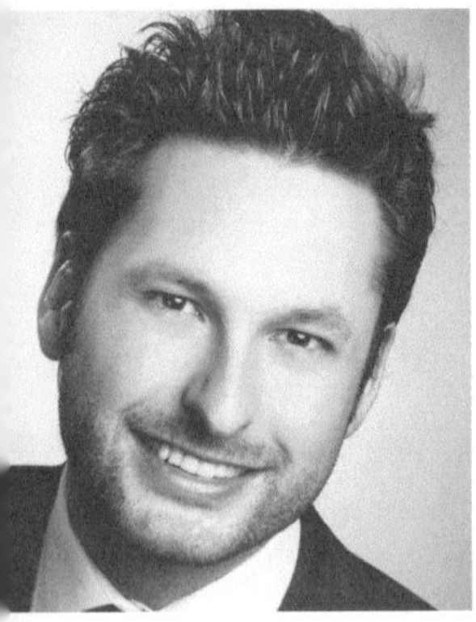
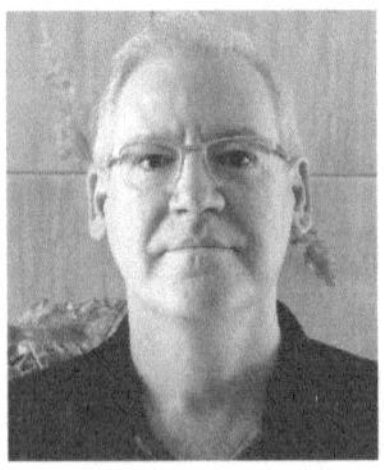

IntechOpen

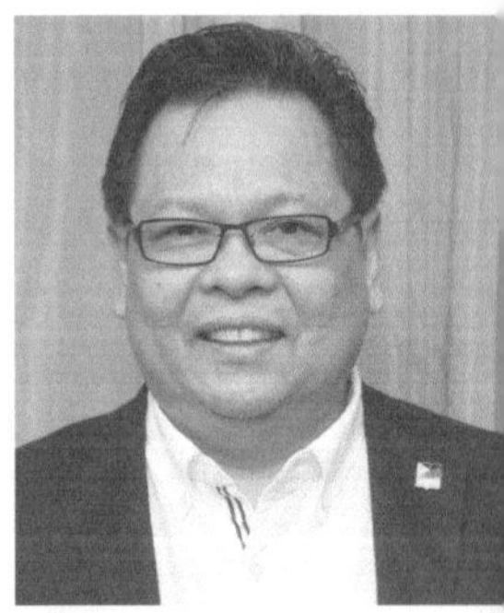
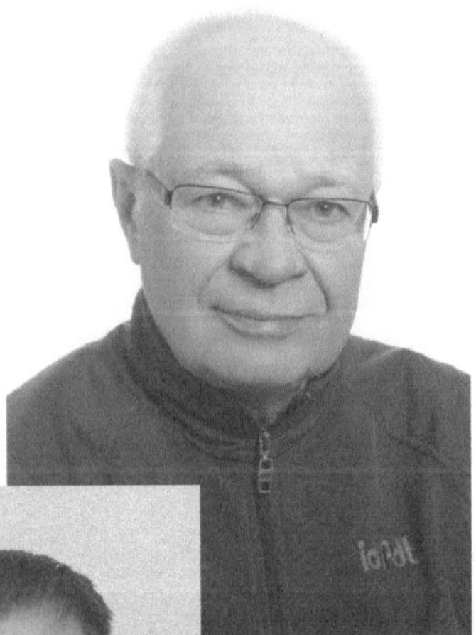
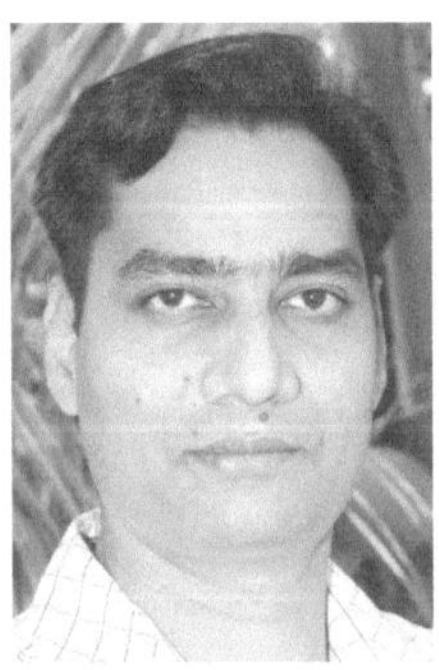
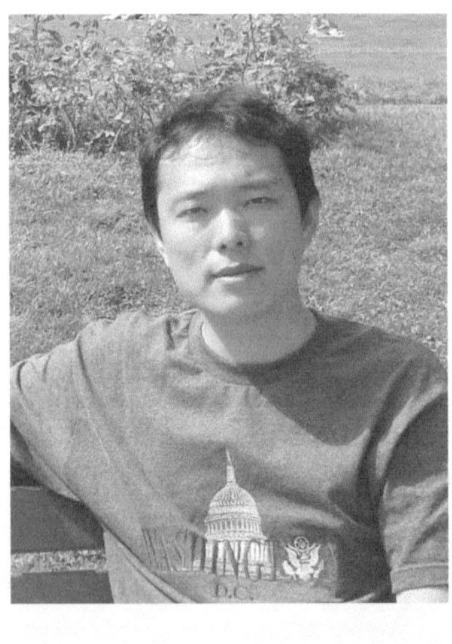
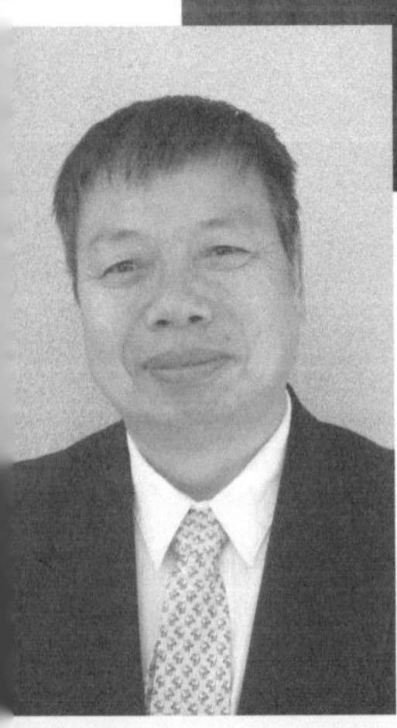
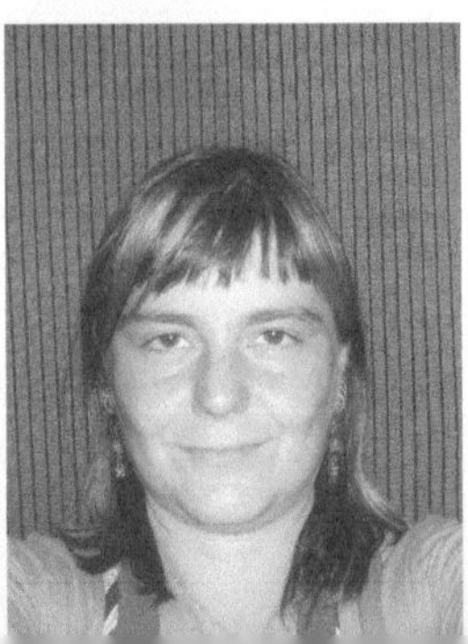

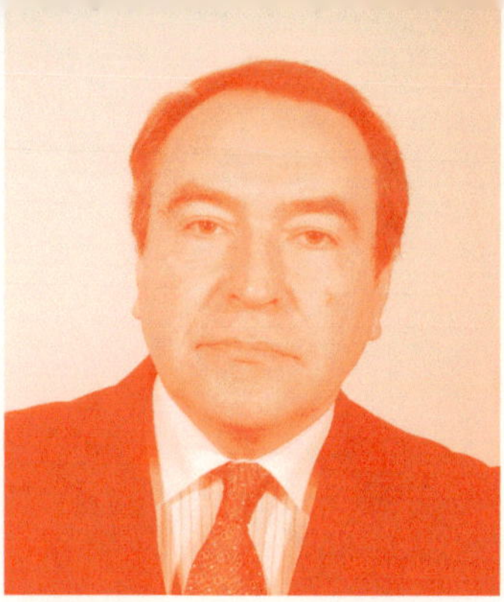
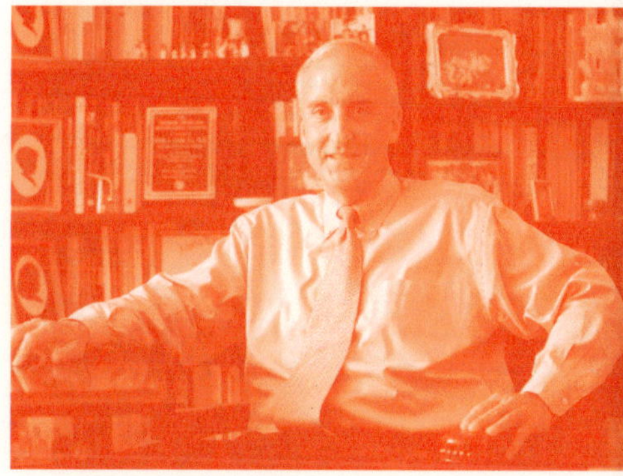
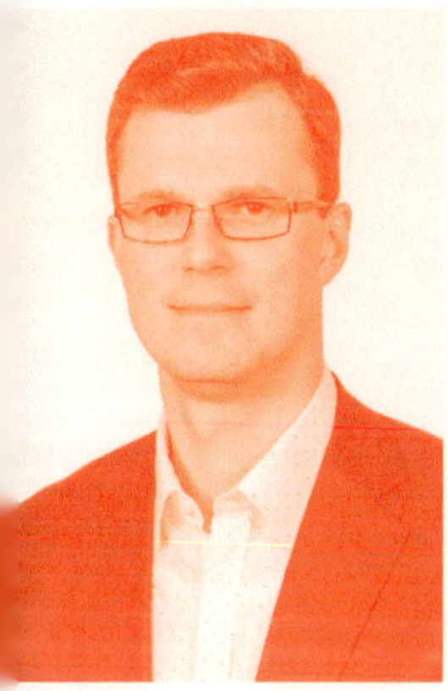
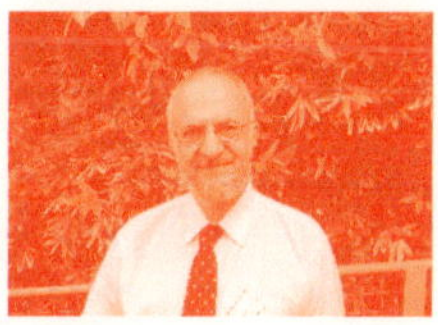
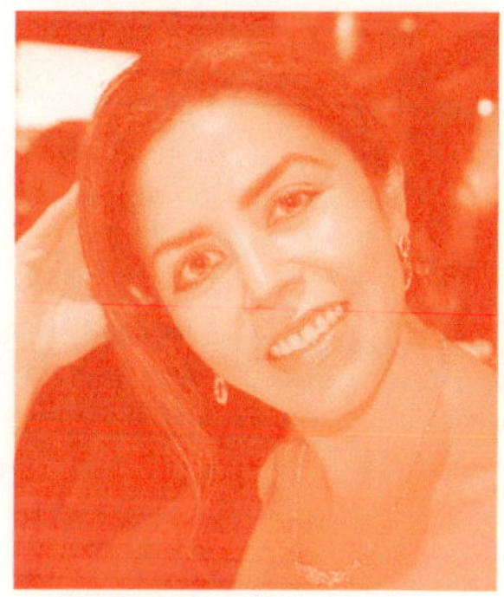

Supporting open minds since 2005

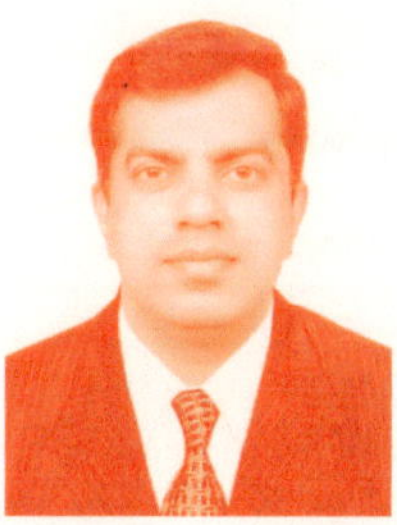
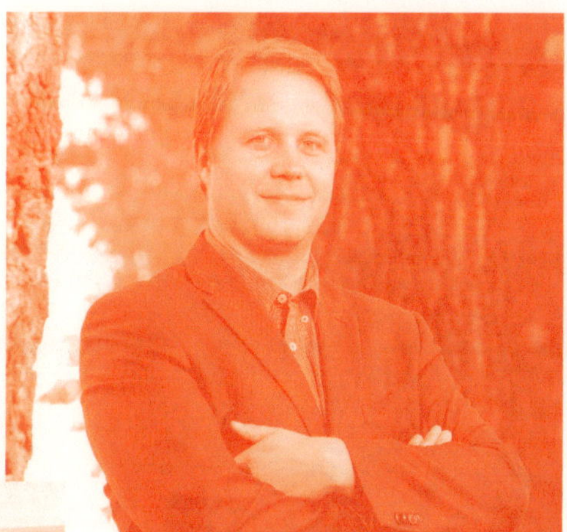
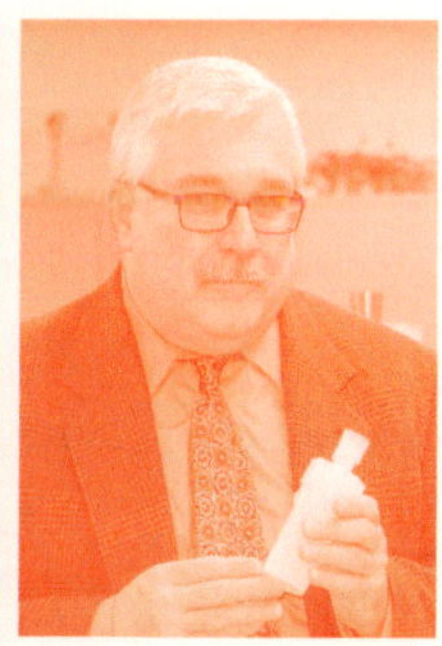
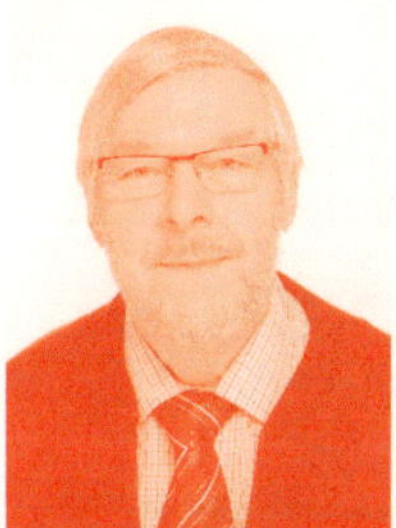
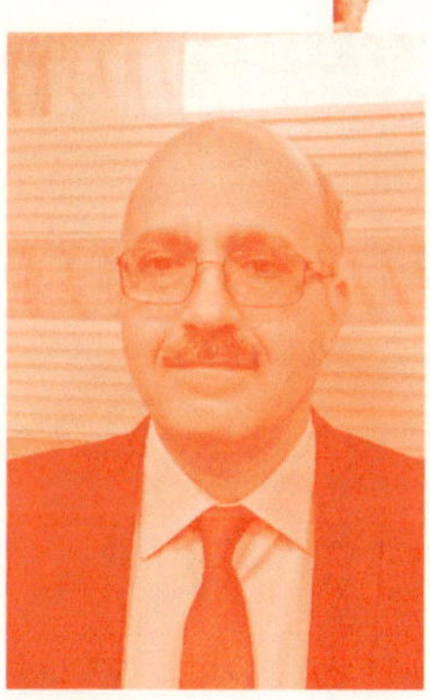
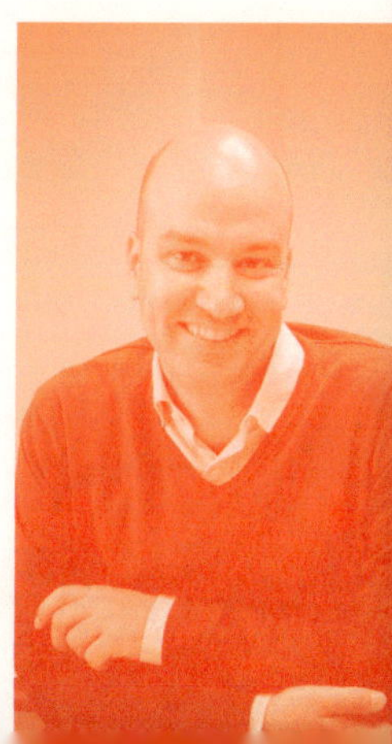
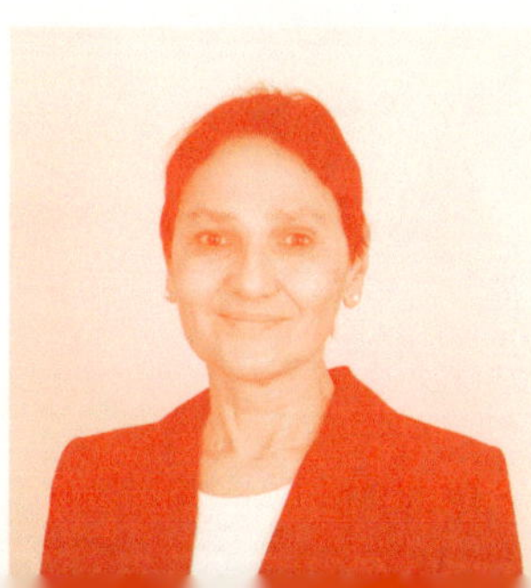

Germ Line Mutations Associated Leukemia
http://dx.doi.org/10.5772/intechopen.77693
Edited by Zhan He Wu

Contributors
Arturo Solis Herrera, Jakub Trizuljak, Michael Doubek, Duohui Jing, Bingzhi He, Julia Cathryn Hlavka-Zhang, Richard B Lock, Zhan He Wu

First published in London, United Kingdom, 2019 by IntechOpen
IntechOpen is the global imprint of INTECHOPEN LIMITED, registered in England and Wales, registration number: 11086078, The Shard, 25th floor, 32 London Bridge Street
London, SE19SG - United Kingdom
Printed in Croatia

British Library Cataloguing-in-Publication Data
A catalogue record for this book is available from the British Library

Additional hard and PDF copies can be obtained from orders@intechopen.com

Germ Line Mutations Associated Leukemia
Edited by Zhan He Wu
p. cm.
Print ISBN 978-1-78984-023-0
Online ISBN 978-1-78984-024-7
eBook (PDF) ISBN 978-1-78984-403-0

Meet the editor

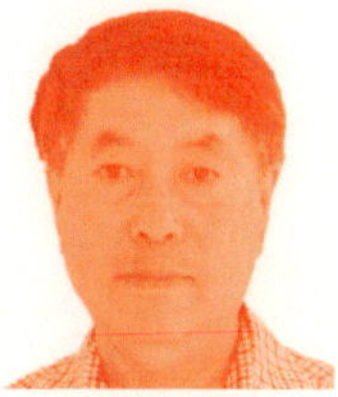

Dr. Zhan He Wu graduated from Harbin Medical University, China, and received his Master's degree in 1985 from the same university. He received his PhD degree in 1993 from the University of New South Wales, Australia.

Since 1996, he has been working in the field of human genetic disease studies in the Sydney Genome Diagnostics, Western Sydney Genetics Program, The Children's Hospital Westmead, Affiliated to the University of Sydney, mainly on hematological malignancies such as leukemia and lymphoma, and inherited bone marrow failure syndromes, including Fanconi anemia (it is named as the prone cancer syndrome and paradigm for cancer and aging research).

Dr. Zhan He Wu has published more than 60 original articles, more than 60 scientific conference presentations, and five chapters in books. He was granted as a Founding Fellow of Royal College of Pathologist for Australasia in 2011. In the past he has organized many national scientific conferences. He was invited as the Chair for the Euro-Global Conference on Pediatrics and Neonatology 2018, 13–15, SEP, ROME, and delivered the welcome message as well. He has been involved in medical journal reviewing and editing and invited by nine international journals as reviewer, associate editor, guest editor, editor, column chair, and so on. Currently, he is editing two professional books in English for a UK publisher: *Germ Line Mutations Associated Leukemia* and *Rare Diseases*.

Contents

Preface

Evidence obtained from studies over the last decade has demonstrated that some types of hematological malignancies, commonly in acute myeloid leukemia and myelodysplastic syndrome, are associated with germ line mutations either in specific gene mutations or genetic-based syndromes, as described and classified officially by the World Health Organization (WHO) in their book *WHO Classification of Tumors of Haematopoietic and Lymphoid Tissues*, 2016.

The four edited chapters in this book are specific to our aim of increasing the awareness, minimizing the underdiagnosis and even misdiagnosis, preventing the occurrence of secondary malignancies, and providing the appropriate treatment strategies for germ line mutations-associated leukemia. This includes the selection of donors for stem cell transplantation and also care for members of affected families by the application of modern technologies. This is because germ line mutations-associated leukemia presents different genetic landscapes and more importantly it requires different therapeutical strategies due to the nature and complexity of the disease. We hope this book will help in the understanding of germ line mutations-associated disease, particularly in leukemogenesis caused by somatic mutations.

Books published on the topic of somatic mutations-associated leukemia are very common, but to our knowledge books published on the topic of germ line mutations-associated leukemia are extremely rare, so far. We all are facing huge challenges but also exciting opportunities in such a special field.

We would like to express our thanks for the contributions from all the experienced authors as follows:

Epigenetics is the concept of genetic functional modification and plays a very important biological role in the control of gene expression without changing the DNA sequence. Studies have found that epigenetics is associated with cancer. Dr. Duohui Jing, Dr. Richard B Lock, Dr. Julia Cathryn Hlavka-Zhang, and Dr. Bingzhi He have contributed their chapter "Epigenetic Landscape in Leukemia and Its Impact on Antileukemia Therapeutics" in which they discuss their novel findings obtained from first-hand studies on the mechanism of therapeutical resistance from specific epigenetic modification.

As mentioned above, WHO has specifically described and classified the myeloid neoplasmas with germ line predisposition and pre-existing platelet disorders. Dr. Jakub Trizuljak and Dr. Michael Doubek have contributed their chapter "Familial Leukemia Associated with Thrombocytopenia" by discussing the association of familial/inherited platelet disorders with germ line mutations-associated leukemia.

Dr. Arturo Solis Herrera has contributed his chapter "Perturbations in Generation and Flow of Energy in the Eukaryotic Cell Explain the Chromosomal Instability Syndrome" from different fields and directions to discuss the association of the pathological mechanism of leukemia.

We also would like to thank the Author Service Manager, Ms. Sandra Maljavac, for her skillful organization and great efforts.

Zhan He Wu
Sydney Genome Diagnostics,
Western Sydney Genetics Program,
The Children's Hospital at Westmead,
Affiliated to the University of Sydney,
Australia

Section 1

Introduction

Chapter 1

Introductory Chapter: Germline Mutations Associated with Leukaemia - Different Genetic Landscape and Therapeutic Strategies

Zhan He Wu

1. Introduction

Dr. Barbara McClintock, the 1983 Nobel Prize winner in physiology or medicine, described that "the most remarkable kinds of mutations are not (usually) produced by such extrinsic factors as radiation and chemicals, but by factors that are intrinsic to the cells themselves".

Evidences obtained from studies proved that genomic mutations are the direct root causes of increased susceptibility to almost all disorders/diseases in the manner of either somatic or germline mutations. Diseases associated with somatic mutations have been well studied; in contrast, studies on diseases associated with germline mutations have been just started, particularly in malignancies.

The estimation by 2015 showed that there were about 17.5 million cancer cases and 8.7 million deaths worldwide per annum [1]. Cancer is a genetic disease caused by mutations from environmental and genetic factors and their interactions. Genetic factors include somatic (acquired) and germline: the difference between germline and somatic mutations is that the germline mutation occurring in reproductive cells (sperm, egg) inherits to the offspring, whereas somatic mutation occurring in body cells is not inherent to the offspring.

In the recent years, more and more attention has been paid to the studies on cancers associated with germline mutations, and more and more discoveries have been achieved by increasing the recognition of such disease. TP53 was the typical and most commonly germline-mutated gene associated with Li-Fraumeni syndrome (colorectal cancer). Studies from Zhang group showed that the rate of germline mutation in cancer-predisposition genes was 8.5%. They estimated that in the hereditary breast/ovarian cancer (HBOC) from BRCA1 and BRAC2 mutations, women with BRCA1 mutations have a 47–66% chance of developing breast cancer and a 35–46% chance of developing ovarian cancer by the age of 70 years [2].

Leukaemia is a type of haematological malignancy (liquid cancer) occurring in haematopoietic tissue caused by environmental and genetic factors, such as other types of cancers, typically presented with fever, bleeding, infection, bone pain and anaemia. The presentation can vary, however, depending on the many different factors of individuals. Among all leukaemia types of the myeloid malignancies, acute myeloid leukaemia (AML), myelodysplastic syndrome (MDS) and chronic myeloid leukaemia (CML) are the common types.

IntechOpen

In a similar scenario with germline mutations associated with solid cancers, about 5–10% of some particular germline mutations will develop to haematological malignancies including MDS, MDS/myeloproliferative neoplasms (MPN) and AML. Germline predisposition of myeloid malignancies is estimated at about 5–10% in the genetic manner, either from functional haplo-insufficiency due to loss of an allele or gain of oncogenic function, but the loss of an allele is more common than gain of oncogenic function in such a type of leukaemia [3].

Studies showed that myeloid neoplasms associated with predisposing of germline mutations are found to be more common than was thought. But it is still under-investigated, under-diagnosed and under-reported due to the low case numbers and nature of disease complexity.

2. Understanding of the WHO's germline mutations associated with neoplasms from gene mutations and syndromes

To increase the recognition for germline predisposition, the major changes were made in the 2016 version of the book *WHO Classification of Tumours of Haematopoietic and Lymphoid Tissues* for the myeloid neoplasms, with the addition of germline predisposition of the myeloid neoplasms under the following categories [4, 5]:

The first category is myeloid neoplasms with germline predisposition without a pre-existing disorder or organ dysfunction with CEBPA and DDX41 mutations.

CCAAT enhancer-binding protein alpha (CEBPA) is involved in the function of myeloid differentiation by encoding a granulocyte differentiation factor located on chromosome 19q13.1. This germline mutation associated with AML is due to the inheritance of a single copy of mutated CEBPA, and studies suggested such mutation has a favourable prognosis than somatic mutation AML [6, 7].

DEAD-Box Helicase (DDX41) is located on chromosome 5q35.3, and studies found that in about 1.5% of myeloid neoplasms, half of these patients had germline mutations, typically in MDS and AML combined with additional del(5q) presented with erythroid dysplasia, leading to erythroid leukaemia with poor prognosis. CML, CMML and lymphomas have been also reported [8, 9].

The second category is myeloid neoplasms with germline predisposition and pre-existing platelet disorders with RUNX1, ANKRD26 and ETV6 mutations.

Runt-related transcription factor 1 (RUNX1, located on chromosome 21q.12) is playing a physiological role in haematopoiesis. RUNX1 mutations cause familial platelet disorder and develop to MDS/AML in 11–100% risk, median 44% [10, 11].

Ankyrin repeat domain-containing protein 26 (ANKRD26, located on chromosome 10p12.1) mutation is characterised by thrombocytopenia from the abnormal megakaryopoiesis and increases risk to MDS and AML in about 30 fold [12, 13].

ETS variant gene 6 (ETV6, located on chromosome 12p13.2) is functional as a haematopoietic regulator in normal physiological condition. ETV6 mutations were found to be associated with several types of haematological malignancies including MDS, AML, B-cell leukaemia and multiple myeloma (MM) as have been identified [14–17].

The third category is the myeloid neoplasms with germline predisposition and other organ dysfunctions with GATA2 mutations and several types of genetic-based syndromes including myeloid neoplasms associated with telomere biology disorders, juvenile myelomonocytic leukaemia associated with neurofibromatosis, Noonan syndrome or Noonan syndrome-like disorders and myeloid neoplasms associated with Down syndrome.

GATA-binding protein 2 (GATA2, located on chromosome 3q21.3) mutations were found to be associated with some syndromes, including MonoMac syndrome, dendritic cell, monocyte, B and NK cell deficiency, familial MDS and Emberger syndrome and some types of disorders such as congenital neutropenia and aplastic anaemia. The risk of developing MDS/AML from GATA2 germline mutations is increased by 70% [18, 19, 20, 21].

3. Germline mutations associated with haematological malignancies in myeloid and lymphoid leukaemias

Most of the findings of germline mutations associated with leukaemia were from myeloid neoplasms. Recent studies found that lymphoid malignancies in acute lymphoblastic leukaemia (ALL) and chronic lymphocytic leukaemia (CLL) are associated with germline mutations. Speedy et al. demonstrated the existence of germline mutations associated with familial CLL by using whole-exome sequencing of 66 CLL families and identified 4 families where loss-of-function mutations in protection of telomeres 1 (POT1) co-segregated with CLL [22]. Qian group studied the loss-of-function germline TP53 variants, and their results suggested that such mutations lead to predispose children to ALL and with adverse treatment outcomes with ALL therapy and increase the risk of second malignant neoplasms [23]. Chang et al. have identified germline mutations from congenital ALL by using the exome sequencing technology [24].

Studies showed that some more genetic-based cancer-prone syndromes with specific germline predisposition syndromes and multiple-cancer hereditary predisposition syndromes are all at an increased risk for haematologic malignancies, commonly in AML, including chromosomal instability syndromes (CIS) such as Nijmegen breakage syndrome, Ataxia telangiectasia, Ataxia telangiectasia-like disorder and Bloom syndrome and including inherited bone marrow failure syndromes (IBMFS) such as dyskeratosis congenita, Shwachman-Diamond syndrome, Diamond-Blackfan anaemia, congenital amegakaryocytic thrombocytopenia, severe congenital neutropenia and thrombocytopenia-absent radii [25].

The most representative example is the Fanconi anaemia (FA) with germline mutations and predisposition to leukaemia. It overlaps in both CIS and IBMFS in its phenotypes. Historically, it was first recognised as a cause of juvenile leukaemia in 1967 [26]. FA is a hereditary disorder with defects in DNA repair and is characterised with multiple gene mutations, multiple types of genetic abnormalities, multiple organ involvements and multiple types of cancer risks [27, 28]. So far, 22 genes responsible for FA have been identified, 4 of them are genes found in breast cancer and some genes were found to be associated with other types of cancers as well.

Patients with FA have very high susceptibility to both haematologic and non-haematologic malignancies. The risk of developing AML and MDS is increased to 785 fold, and the median age of patients developing to AML is 14 years. AML occurs at about 9% and MDS is about 7% of all patients with FA, respectively [29]. Cells from FA patient associated with leukaemia showed high sensitive reaction to chemotherapies than non-FA patient with leukaemia.

FA was the first successful remarkable milestone in cord blood stem cell transplantation in 1988. The studies on FA offered insights into the pathogenesis of many types of human diseases, particularly in non-genetic bone marrow failure, ageing and cancer. So the study on FA is named as a paradigm for the understanding of cancer and ageing.

In the last couple of years, studies, by using the modern genetic technologies particularly by the next-generation sequencing (NGS) approach to study known and new germline mutations in familial acute myeloid leukaemia and myelodysplastic syndromes, found more leukaemia predisposition genes associated with germ line in variants in cancer-predisposition genes, mainly as ASXL1, BCOR, NRAS,

TP53, CEBPA, FLT3, EZH2, IDH1, IDH2, NPM1, DNMT3A, TET2, CBL, KRAS, SF3B1, SRSF2, U2AF1, ZRSR2, TERT, TERC and SRP72 [30–32]. Studies from Seiter group provided the direct evidence from ASXL1 germline mutation associated with leukaemia studied on father and son [33]. Buijs et al. defined CBFA2 single-nucleotide mutation in a familial leukaemia [34].

Recommendations and guides are available by the applications of the next-generation sequencing approaches (NGS) [35, 36]. Churpek et al. proposed recommendations on the screening, identification, genetic counselling and managements on inherited susceptibility to MDS and acute leukaemia [37].

4. Conclusion

To increase the awareness and recognition for germline mutations associated with leukaemia is extremely important and imperative in the clinical practice by performing the specific tests. The significances are (1) to diagnose such type of patients earlier even if before the occurrence of such type of leukaemia, (2) to prevent the occurrence of secondary cancers, (3) to care other members of the family, (4) to design a specific therapeutical strategy, personalised medicine and long-term follow-up and (5) to guide the selection of donors for patient bone marrow stem cell transplantation.

To study germline mutations and syndromes associated with leukaemia has provided exciting and significant opportunities with such new discoveries. The studies on germline mutations associated with leukaemia will not only be useful in its clinical diagnosis, classification, stratification and specific treatment strategies, but it will also provide an insight to understand human diseases, such as tumorigenesis, particularly in somatic mutations associated with leukemogenesis. It is certainly that more and more such disorders will be identified in the future.

The huge challenges are to identify germline mutation associated with leukaemia due to the lack of awareness and knowledge about these disorders, lack of at least easy and practical available testing methods and sufficient familial history of individuals and lack of specimen source to represent genome for these individuals. The complex and mysterious genetic variation is another challenging issue just as the English novelist, George Orwell, described that "all cancer is genetic, but some cancers are more genetic than others which it hinted the mechanism and genetic variations of cancers".

Author details

Zhan He Wu
Sydney Genome Diagnostics, Western Sydney Genetics Program, The Children's Hospital at Westmead, NSW, Australia

*Address all correspondence to: zhan.wu@health.nsw.gov.au.

References

[1] Fitzmaurice C. Global, regional, and national cancer incidence, mortality, years of life lost, years lived with disability, and disability-adjusted life-years for 32 cancer groups, 1990 to 2015, a systematic analysis for the global burden of disease study. JAMA Oncology. 2017;**3**(4):524-548

[2] Ngeow J, Eng C. Precision medicine in heritable cancer: When somatic tumour testing and germline mutations meet. NPJ Genomic Medicine. 2016;**1**:1-3

[3] Zhang JH, Walsh MF, Wu G, et al. Germline mutations in predisposition genes in pediatric cancer. The New England Journal of Medicine. 2015;**373**:2336-2346

[4] Swerdlow SH, Campo E, Harris NL, et al. WHO Classification of Tumours of Haematopoietic and Lymphoid Tissues, Revised. 4th ed. Vol. 22017. International Agency for Research on Cancer. Lyon, France; pp. 121-128

[5] Arber DA, Orazi A, Hasserjian R, et al. The 2016 revision to the World Health Organization classification of myeloid neoplasms and acute leukemia. Blood. 2016;**127**(20):2391-2405

[6] Godley LA. Inherited predisposition to acute myeloid leukemia. Seminars in Hematology. 2014;**51**(4):306-321

[7] Pabst T, Eyholzer M, Fos J, et al. Heterogeneity within AML with CEBPA mutations; only CEBPA double mutations, but not single CEBPA mutations are associated with favourable prognosis. British Journal of Cancer. 2009;**100**:1343-1346

[8] West AH, Godley LA, Churpek JE. Familial myelodysplastic syndrome/ acute leukemia syndromes: A review and utility for translational investigations. Annals of the New York Academy of Sciences. 2014;**1310**:111-118

[9] Bannon SA, DiNardo CD. Hereditary predispositions to myelodysplastic syndrome. International Journal of Molecular Sciences. 2016;**17**:2-11

[10] Owen CJ, Toze CL, Anna Koochin A, et al. Five new pedigrees with inherited RUNX1 mutations causing familial platelet disorder with propensity to myeloid malignancy. Blood. 2008;(12):4639-4645

[11] Bellissimo DC, Speck NA. RUNX1 mutations in inherited and sporadic leukemia. Frontiers in Cell and Developmental Biology. 2017;**5**(111):1-11

[12] Noris P, Perrotta S, Seri M, et al. Mutations in ANKRD26 are responsible for a frequent form of inherited thrombocytopenia: Analysis of 78 patients from 21 families. Blood. 2011;**117**:6673-6680

[13] Noris P, Favier R, Alessi MC, et al. ANKRD26-related thrombocytopenia and myeloid malignancies. Blood. 2013;**122**:1987-1989

[14] Zhang MY, Churpek JE, Keel SB, et al. Germline ETV6 mutations in familial thrombocytopenia and hematologic malignancy. Nature Genetics. 2015;**47**(2):180-185

[15] Noetzli L, Lo RW, Lee-Sherick AB, et al. Germline mutations in ETV6 are associated with thrombocytopenia, red cell macrocytosis and predisposition to lymphoblastic leukemia. Nature Genetics. 2015;**47**(5):535-538

[16] Topka S, Vijai J, Walsh MF, et al. Germline ETV6 mutations confer susceptibility to acute lymphoblastic leukemia and thrombocytopenia. PLoS Genetics. 2015;**11**(6):1-14

[17] Moriyama T, Metzger ML, Wu G, et al. Germline genetic variation in

ETV6 and risk of childhood acute lymphoblastic leukaemia: A systematic genetic study. The Lancet Oncology. 2015;**16**(16):1659-1666

[18] Hahn CN, Chong CE, Carmichael CL, et al. Heritable GATA2 mutations associated with familial myelodysplastic syndrome and acute myeloid leukemia. Nature Genetics. 2011;**43**(10):1012-1017

[19] Ostergaard P, Simpson MA Connell FC, et al. Mutations in GATA2 cause primary lymphedema associated with a predisposition to acute myeloid leukemia (Emberger syndrome). Nature Genetics. 2011;**43**:929-931

[20] Micol JB, Abdel-Wahab O. ASXL1 mutations in patients with germline GATA2 mutations. Haematologica. 2014;**99**(2):201-203

[21] Mateos MK, Barbaric D, Sally-Anne Byatt SA, et al. Down syndrome and leukemia: Insights into leukemogenesis and translational targets. Translational Pediatrics. 2015;**4**(2):76-92

[22] Speedy HE, Kinnersley B, Chubb D, et al. Germline mutations in shelterin complex genes are associated with familial chronic lymphocytic leukemia. Blood. 2016;**128**(19):2319-2326

[23] Qian M, Cao X, Devidas M, et al. TP53 germline variations influence the predisposition and prognosis of B-cell acute lymphoblastic leukemia in children. Journal of Clinical Oncology. 2018;**36**:591-599

[24] Chang CY, Basso G, Sakamoto KM, et al. Identification of somatic and germline mutations using whole exome sequencing of congenital acute lymphoblastic leukemia. BMC Cancer. 2013;**13**:55

[25] Wu ZH. Inherited bone marrow failure and chromosome instability syndromes and their cancer predisposition. In: Hassan, editor. Contemporary Pediatric Hematology and Oncology. UK: IntechOpen; 2019. pp. 1-20

[26] Fanconi G. Familiäre infantile perniziosaartige Anämie (perniziöses Blutbild und Konstitution). Jahrb Kinderh. 1927;**117**:257-280

[27] Wu ZH. The concept and practice of Fanconi anemia: From the clinical bedside to the laboratory bench. Translational Pediatrics. 2013;**2**(3):112-119

[28] Rosenberg P, Greene MH, Alter BP. Cancer incidence in persons with Fanconi anemia. Blood. 2003;**101**:822-826

[29] Alter BP. Cancer in Fanconi anemia 1927-2001. Cancer. 2003;**97**:425-440

[30] Kirwan M, Walne AJ, Plagnol V, et al. Exome sequencing identifies autosomal-dominant SRP72 mutations associated with familial aplasia and myelodysplasia. The American Journal of Human Genetics. 2012;**90**:888-892

[31] Döhner H, Estey E, Grimwade D, et al. Diagnosis and management of AML in adults. ELN recommendations from an international expert panel. Blood. 2017;**129**(4):424-447

[32] Rocquain J, Carbuccia N, Trouplin V, et al. Combined mutations of ASXL1, CBL, FLT3, IDH1, IDH2, JAK2, KRAS, NPM1, NRAS, RUNX1, TET2 and WT1 genes in myelodysplastic syndromes and acute myeloid leukemias. BMC Cancer. 2010;**10**:401. DOI: 10.1186/1471-2407-10-401

[33] Seiter K, Htun K, Baskind P, et al. Acute myeloid leukemia in a father and son with a germline mutation of ASXL1. Biomarker Research. 2018;**6**:7. DOI: 10.1186/s40364-018-0121-3

[34] Buijs A, Poddighe P, van Wijk R, et al. A novel CBFA2 single-nucleotide

mutation in familial platelet disorder with propensity to develop myeloid malignancies. Blood. 2001;**98**:2856-2858

[35] Hussaini MO, Mirza A-S, Komrokji R et al. Genetic Landscape of Acute Myeloid Leukemia Interrogated by Next-generation Sequencing: A Large Cancer Center Experience. Cancer Genomics & Proteomics. 2018;**15**:121-126

[36] The University of Chicago Hematopoietic Malignancies Cancer Risk Team. How I diagnose and manage individuals at risk for inherited myeloid malignancies. Blood. 2016;**128**:1800-1813

[37] Churpek JE, Lorenz R, Nedumgottil S, et al. Proposal for the clinical detection and management of patients and their family members with familial myelodysplastic syndrome/acute leukemia predisposition syndromes. Leukemia & Lymphoma. 2013;**54**:28-35

Section 2

Epigenetic Mechanisms Associated Leukemia

Chapter 2

Epigenetic Landscape in Leukemia and Its Impact on Antileukemia Therapeutics

Bingzhi He, Julia Cathryn Hlavka-Zhang, Richard B. Lock and Duohui Jing

Abstract

Epigenomic landscape mapping in leukemia cells supports germ line mutation studies to understand pathogenicity and treatment plans. The differential regulation of gene expression and heterogeneity between cell types during hematopoiesis and leukemia development is important in understanding oncogenesis. Oncogenesis in leukemia occurs at both genomic and epigenomic levels in order for hematological cells to evade lineage commitment. To ensure that therapies target the entire malignancy, it is important to consider the regulatory network that drives malignancy caused by mutations. Therapies tailored to respond to a patient-specific epigenetic landscape have the potential to minimize risk in administering chemotherapies that may not work. In this chapter, a focused study on childhood acute lymphoblastic leukemia (ALL) will be used as an example of the current research in the field of epigenetics in leukemia and the impact it carries on our understanding of the disease and treatment plans.

Keywords: epigenome, childhood acute lymphoblastic leukemia, chemotherapy, glucocorticoid, epigenetic drugs

1. Epigenetics overview

Epigenetics is a biological system that describes phenotypes and occurs due to differential regulation of genes (as opposed to genetic mutations). Current epigenetic studies include the control of basic biological functions [1], developmental biology [2, 3], the origin of disease [4], and cancer therapeutics [5]. Investigating the regulatory mechanisms driving these results involves genome-wide mapping of chromatin accessibility and conformation, transcription factor (TF) binding, DNA methylation, and histone modifications. Leukemia oncogenesis is a result of both genetic and epigenetic factors, whereby hematopoietic pathways are disrupted and leukemia cells are able to evade lineage commitment. This interdependence between altered genes and gene regulation is critical in cancer development. Consequently, a broader understanding inclusive of genomics and epigenomics will allow for development of drug targets which may limit cancer progression, improve therapeutic response, and find novel targeted therapies.

1.1 Regulation of gene expression

Multicellular eukaryotic organisms consist of a complex variety of different cells, all containing identical genomic DNA. The ability to create such diversity from identical duplicates of DNA is attributed to differential gene expression regulation. Gene expression is as product of epigenetic regulatory systems. Differences within these regulations result in differential expressions and subsequently, cell types that differ in structure and function [6].

The three-dimensional organization of DNA is central to gene expression, as it depends on physical access to the gene to be expressed. Genomic DNA is condensed and wrapped around histone proteins, forming chromatin [7]. Condensed chromatin structures inhibit gene transcription by making the gene physically inaccessible for transcriptional machinery to access (**Figure 1**). To unfold chromatin structure and expose the gene for transcription, endogenous mechanisms and drugs modify the histone proteins around which the DNA is bound [8, 9]. Modifications which result in gene silencing include histone deacetylation and DNA methylation. To achieve differential expression profiles between cell types, cells have different gene access profiles controlled by protein mediation, external stimuli, and development of cells [10].

1.1.1 Histone deacetylation

Histone deacetylation involves the switching of histone proteins from a positive to neutral charge via the addition of an acetyl to a lysine residue within the histone tail. This change in charge will result in the DNA (negatively charged) separation from the histone due to repulsion forces of like charges. Separated DNA regions become accessible to transcriptional machinery as a result. When this mechanism is reversed and lysines are deacetylated, DNA is attracted back toward the protein, resulting in tight DNA wrapping, thus inaccessible for transcriptional machinery (**Figure 2**) [11]. The enzyme responsible for acetylation of histone proteins is called histone acetyltransferase (HAT), which opens the chromatin structure and allows transcription. Deacetylating enzymes which cause compacting of chromatin are called histone deacetylases (HDAC).

1.1.2 DNA methylation

DNA methylation is another mechanism of chromatin remodeling. CpG islands are target sites in the genome for methylation by the DNA methyltransferase

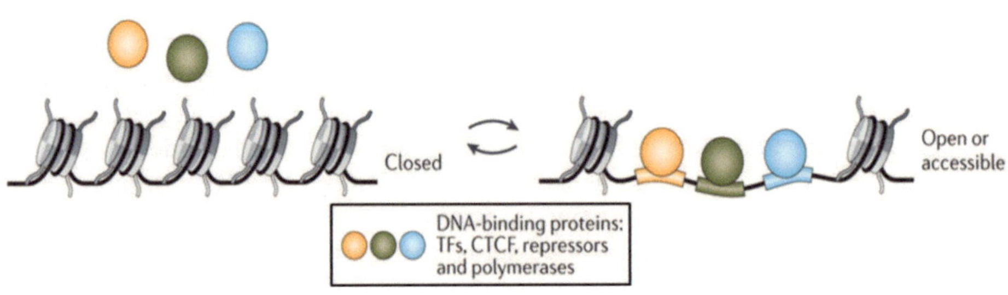

Figure 1.
Chromatin accessibility. Chromatin accessibility modulates gene expression. Densely packed chromatin (left) is inaccessible, preventing transcription factors (TFs), CCCTC-binding factor (CTCF), and polymerases from binding and subsequent gene expression. Opened chromatin structure (right) can be accessed by TFs, CTCF, and polymerases bindings, resulting in ability for gene transcription. Opened and closed chromatin structures are regulated by the acetylation status of histone proteins. Acetylated histones provide an open chromatin structure, while deacetylated histones form a closed chromatin structure. Adapted from Shlyueva et al., 2014 [10].

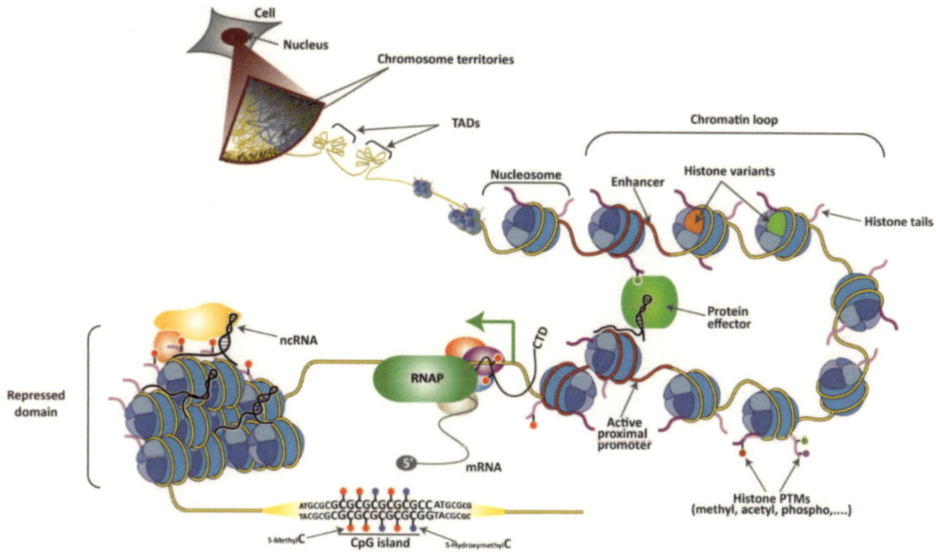

Figure 2.
Hierarchical layers of chromatin organization in mammalian cells. Adapted from Aranda et al., 2015 [11].

(DNMT) enzyme. Of the CpG sites in gene promoter regions, 70% are primary targets for methylation. DNMT prevents gene transcription via physically preventing transcription factor binding and by methylating DNA. Methylated DNA binds to methyl-CpG-binding domain (MBD) proteins that in turn recruit proteins such as histone deacetylase and other chromatin-remodeling proteins. In this new environment, chromatin becomes compact and inactive, termed heterochromatin (repressed domain in **Figure 2**).

1.2 Epigenetics in leukemia

ALL population studies indicated a trend in disease peak around the age of 5, after which there is no increase in prevalence (**Figure 3**). Evidences suggest hematopoietic regulatory network probably most highly involved in leukemia development at their highest in children <5 years old. Case-control studies have shown that the occurrence of childhood ALL is inversely linked to the degree of exposure to infections in the first few months of life [12, 13]. This suggests that there may be certain oncogenic factors present in the early days of a child's life that lead to the development of ALL, rather than being present later on or in adulthood. Addressing these up- and downregulations of oncogenic factors in this critical stage of hematopoiesis will provide insight into pathogenesis and progression of ALL beyond the genetic level.

1.2.1 Oncogenesis driven by epigenetics (in ALL)

Epigenetics is still in the early stages of investigation and translational clinical use. Primary testing in clinics focuses on cytogenic studies, categorizing disease based on genetic abnormalities and cell markers, and then treating the patient accordingly; screening gene expression to map out regulatory profiles of a tumor are less established. In acute lymphoblastic leukemia (ALL), subtypes are diagnosed based on cytogenic testing and testing for markers [14]. In vivo mouse studies, however, have indicated that in almost 75% of diagnosed cases, chromosomal changes alone are insufficient to induce ALL [15]. Investigation of

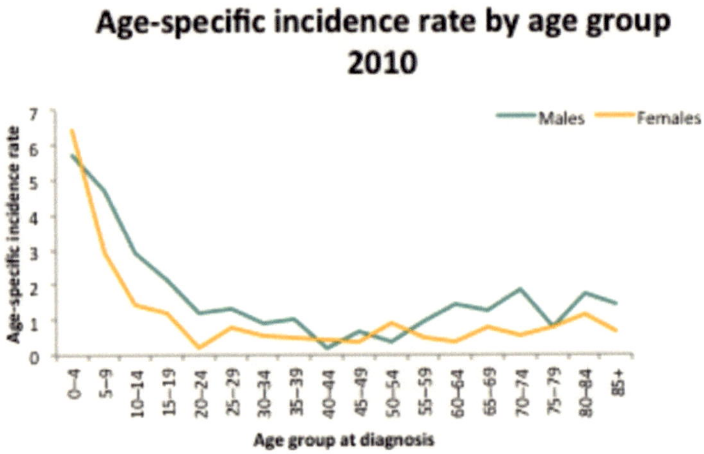

Figure 3.
Incidence of ALL per 100,000 populations in 2010. Source: Australian Institute of Health and Welfare (AIHW), 2014 [97].

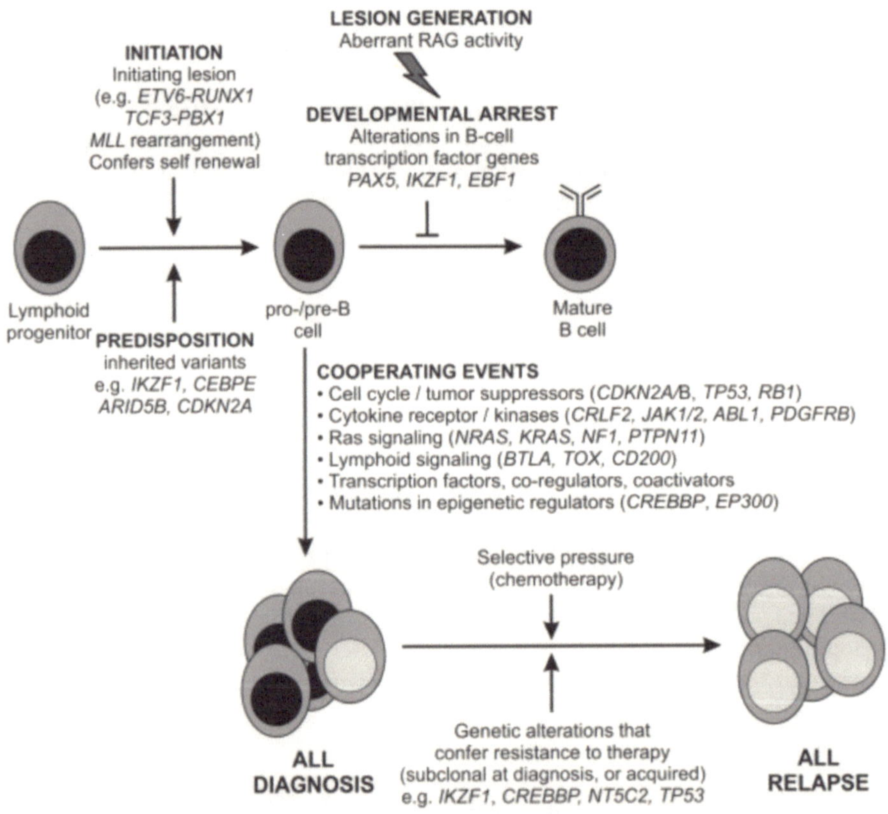

Figure 4.
B-ALL development. Multiple mutations contribute to the development of ALL. Mutations in ALL predisposing genes, e.g., IKZF1, and initiating genes, e.G., ETV6-RUNX1, and MLL rearrangement will promote ALL development. Alterations in B-cell development genes, e.G., PAX5 and IKZF1, inhibit cell maturation, resulting in the accumulation of immature cells. This alone however is not enough to cause ALL pathogenesis. Cell cycle and lymphoid lineage regulatory gene expression must also be altered to promote its survival. Further alterations may induce chemoresistance. Adapted from Mullighan, 2013 [15].

genetic alterations alongside epigenetics microarrays of gene expression suggested an association between mutations and altered regulation in gene expressions during hematopoiesis in both B-ALL and T-ALL [14, 15]. Prenatal lesions and postnatal-acquired mutations have also shown impaired regulation and development of progenitor B cells or T cells [16–18]. Together, these studies suggest that it is not mutations alone that act as oncogenic drivers but also an altered gene regulatory network.

Thus far, ALL oncogenic studies have reported prenatal genetic lesions and inherited genetic predisposition which neither can stand alone to account for the disease. Prenatal genetic lesions have been reported with an unknown pathogenesis [18], and only 5% of ALL patients reported with an inherited genetic predisposition such as Down's syndrome and Bloom's syndrome [17, 19]. **Figure 4** indicates multiple genetic lesions contributing to an altered regulatory network in healthy lymphoid development toward a pathogenic ALL pathway [20–23]. Incomplete evidence regarding prenatal genetic lesions in ALL supports research into the epigenetic regulatory system in the development of ALL. Prenatal genetic lesions suggest the preleukemic states. Despite studies suggesting preleukemic state in utero, other studies show that the development of ALL in monozygotic twins follows a different time course. The difference in postnatal disease progression despite an identical prenatal state suggests the role of epigenetics in ALL manifestation [24–27].

2. Targeting epigenome of ALL in chemotherapy

Since drugs target distinct cell pathways relying on gene expression, access to target genes is crucial for the treatment to work. A common ALL chemotherapy regimen of glucocorticoids relies on activation of the glucocorticoid receptor (GR), which binds to glucocorticoid-response elements (GREs) in gene promoters, to induce expression of pro-apoptotic pathways [28]. Using a DNase hypersensitivity assay (DHA) to determine chromatin accessibility [29], the majority of GR binding to GREs were identified in open chromatin [8, 30]. Thus, glucocorticoid therapy is dependent on GRE accessibility which is defined by chromatin accessibility. Resistance and patient response to such drugs is thought to be dependent on their gene accessibility profiles.

2.1 Glucocorticoid-based chemotherapy: Focused study on ALL

2.1.1 Acute lymphoblastic leukemia (ALL)

ALL is a malignant disease in both adults and children, with mutations developing along the lymphoid lineage starting at the lymphoid progenitor cells. Normally, lymphoid cells have the potential to differentiate into B or T cells, which under oncogenic conditions give rise to either B-ALL or T-ALL [17, 21]. Hematopoietic stem cells (HSCs), in the bone marrow, are the origin of both lymphoid and myeloid lineages. The tight regulation of gene expression in HSCs determines the lineage pathway and development. During oncogenesis, molecular defects and abnormal genes regulation may alter the differentiation of HSC; these factors may also contribute to further alterations downstream in hematopoiesis [17, 31–36]. Alterations along the lymphoid lineage result in abnormal pre-lymphoid cells called lymphoblasts; these aggressively proliferate and gradually replace the normal hematopoietic cells in the bone marrow and blood. Accumulation of lymphoblasts results in immunity retardation due to the insufficient amounts of mature lymphoid cells. Patients thus become immunocompromised and prone to various infectious diseases normally fought off by the immune system's lymphocytes [21, 37, 38].

2.1.2 Glucocorticoids in the clinic

Glucocorticoids are naturally occurring steroid hormones that are widely recognized for their anti-inflammatory and immunosuppressing activities [39–41]. In leukemia, glucocorticoids are able to induce apoptosis in lymphoid cells. As such, glucocorticoid drugs such as dexamethasone and prednisolone are used as part of multi-agent chemotherapy regimens treating hematological malignancies [42–44], including ALL, chronic lymphocytic leukemia, multiple myeloma, and lymphoma. Due to pro-apoptotic pathway activation, glucocorticoids have remained the pivot point in chemotherapy treatment to combat ALL for 50 years [38, 45].

Glucocorticoids play a role in all three phases of treatment phases. During the remission-induction phase, glucocorticoids make up a significant portion of drug when administered in combination with vincristine and asparaginase and/or anthracycline. This initial high glucocorticoid portion aims to relieve at least 99% of the leukemic burden; the patient's response is critical in determining the future course of treatment and determining chance of relapse and prognosis [46]. The following two chemotherapy phases are less intensive, involving re-administration of remission-induction drugs in addition to methotrexate and mercaptopurine [17]. To note, some patients do not need to be administered pulses of glucocorticoids in phases two and three of the therapy, due to patients' contraindications [47]. This three-phase glucocorticoid regimen has seen an increase in ALL 5-year survival rate from 73–90% in the past 20 years [48], yet there still exits a subset of ALL patients who are resistant to glucocorticoids, resulting in poor prognosis.

2.1.3 Glucocorticoid mechanism of action

Glucocorticoid mode of action involves the activation of specific cellular pathways specific in lymphoid cells to induce cell death. Depending on cell type, cell-specific chromatin conformation provides the structural framework for transcription factor (TF) binding to regulate gene transcription that determines the ability of a cell to activate a pathway [49–51]. A cell-type-specific conformation is generated [11, 52] with each type having approximately 70,000–100,000 accessible chromatin domains and a network of cell-type-specific binding of transcriptional regulators [10, 53, 54]. Glucocorticoids are able to target intracellular pathways by interacting with the glucocorticoid receptor (GR) in the cytoplasm [55, 56]. The complex then translocates into the nucleus and binds at accessible chromatin domains containing glucocorticoid-response elements (GREs) at proximal promoter regions and/or distal sites of a gene [57–59]. GR binding to GREs induces chromatin remodeling and activates gene transcription via recruitment of other transcription proteins [60, 61]. To keep gene transcription tightly regulated, GR binding is highly selective and predetermined by chromatin accessibility in different cell types [8, 62]. Currently, the GR-binding landscape in different cell subsets, as well as between glucocorticoid-sensitive and resistant leukemia subsets, is yet to be established. Understanding this epigenetic landscape is crucial in understanding patient relapse or chemoresistance. Preliminary studies have started this investigation in pediatric ALL, to understand the mechanism of drug resistance in B-ALL.

2.1.4 Limitations to glucocorticoid treatment

While the glucocorticoid induces apoptosis pathway is still unclear, it is a pro-apoptotic pathway exclusive to lymphoid cells despite widespread expressions of GR in most human tissues [63, 64]. Glucocorticoids are rarely efficacious in treating myeloid leukemia [65]. Due to this lymphoid-specific apoptosis pathway, it is hypothesized that glucocorticoid-sensitive cells have a distinguished chromatin structure allowing for specific GR binding at GREs that glucocorticoid-resistant lymphoids, myeloid cells, and other tissue cells do not have [8, 66-69]. Therefore, understanding the lymphocyte-specific mechanisms of glucocorticoid-induced apoptosis, as well as the development of resistance to this class of steroid hormones, is critical in optimizing glucocorticoid-based therapies in the clinic.

The actions of glucocorticoids are cell type specific [65–67], although the exact molecular basis for this differential function remained elusive. While certain signaling pathways resulting from ALL oncogenes appear to interfere with glucocorticoid actions resulting in resistance, epigenetic evidence suggests that in addition to genetic alterations, epigenetic factors contribute to resistance. For instance, inhibition of GR expression or its translocation to the nucleus in vitro and in vivo models via *BTG1* or *PTEN* loss can cause glucocorticoid resistance by [70, 71]; however, GR function is rarely blocked in resistant ALL PDXs [72]. Mutations in epigenetic regulators such as *KMT2D*, *CREBBP*, and *HDAC7*, in two of five resistant PDX models, could not account for abnormal epigenetic changes. Mutations in various signaling pathways [73–76] have been reported to impair glucocorticoid-induced apoptosis in ALL by downregulating the GR-activated pro-apoptotic gene, *BIM* expression. The importance to study beyond gene mutations, toward epigenetic mapping of GR binding, will provide a deeper understanding into individual drug response.

2.2 Epigenetic landscape shapes the response to glucocorticoids in leukemia

Lymphocyte-specific enhancers associated with glucocorticoid-induced apoptosis were identified in cell-wide studies [5, 28]. Moreover, aberrations at these enhancers were observed in glucocorticoid-resistant ALL cells. Similarly, nonlymphoid cells also exhibited inaccessible chromatin at these enhancers, providing insights into the cell-type-specific actions of glucocorticoids. A link between epigenetic differences and cell-type-specific actions of glucocorticoids are essential in the treatment determining treatment approaches for lymphoid malignancies. Lymphocyte-specific epigenetic modifications pre-determine glucocorticoid resistance in ALL and may account for the lack of glucocorticoid sensitivity in other cell types. Recent findings suggest that in glucocorticoid-sensitive cells, GR cooperates with the structural protein, CTCF, at lymphocyte-specific regulatory domains to mediate the formation of a transcriptionally active DNA loop to trigger gene transcription, which can be inhibited by increased DNA methylation in glucocorticoid-resistant ALL. By using a comprehensive map of chromatin accessibility, CTCF binding, histone modifications, and DNA methylation in normal and malignant cell types, there is evidence of regulatory heterogeneity in the epigenome of different cell types. Azacytidine, a DNA demethylating drug that is routinely used in the clinic, could partially reverse these changes and restore glucocorticoid-induced gene expression and glucocorticoid sensitivity. This indicates that reversal of epigenetic changes may lead to improvements in the use of glucocorticoids for the management of lymphoid malignancies.

3. Epigenetic drugs

3.1 What are epigenetic drugs?

Epigenetic drugs inhibit and manipulate different epigenetic regulators involved in histone remodeling. Drugs which target epigenetic regulators can open closed chromatin structures commonly found in chemotherapy-resistant patients.

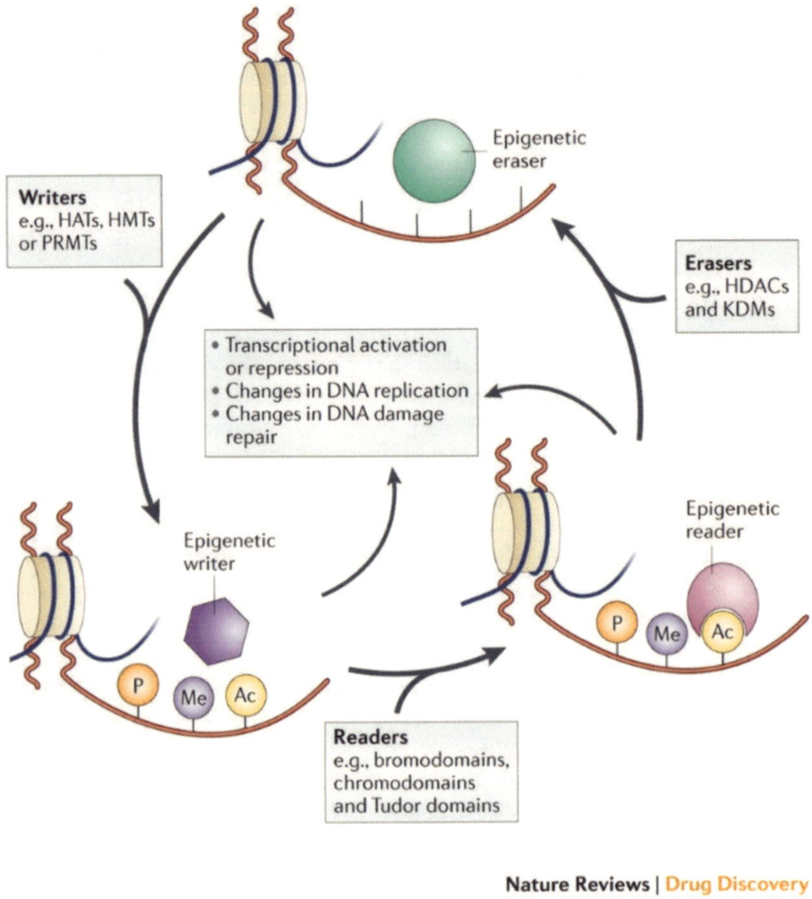

Figure 5.
Epigenetic reader, writer, and eraser. Epigenetic writers such as histone acetyltransferases (HATs), histone methyltransferases (HMTs), protein arginine methyltransferases (PRMTs), and kinases lay down epigenetic marks on amino acid residues on histone tails. Epigenetic readers are proteins that contain bromodomains, chromodomains, and Tudor domains, allowing them to bind to these epigenetic marks. Epigenetic erasers such as histone deacetylases, lysine demethylases, and phosphatases catalyze the removal of epigenetic marks. Together they modulate chromatin structures and regulate various DNA-dependent biological processes such as DNA synthesis and replication. Adapted from Falkenberg and Johnstone, 2014 [77].

Epigenetic regulators can be divided into different categories based on their method of modification: epigenetic writers, readers, and erasers (**Figure 5**).

Epigenetic regulators determine gene expression, and an understanding of them allows for the development of drugs to regulate gene expression over epigenetic marks. Epigenetic writers lay down epigenetic marks on DNA or amino acid residues on histones tails [77]. Examples include histone acetyltransferases (HATs), histone methyltransferases (HMTs), and protein arginine methyltransferases (PRMTs). Drugs which target these are DNA hypomethylating agents, bromodomains, and HDAC inhibitors. Epigenetic readers are proteins that contain bromodomains, chromodomains, and Tudor domains allowing them to bind to specific epigenetic marks on chromatin. Epigenetic erasers such as histone deacetylases, lysine demethylases, and phosphatases catalyze the removal of epigenetic marks.

3.2 Categories of epigenetic modifying drugs

The epigenetic drugs to be discussed are designed to target different epigenetic regulators responsible for gene silencing.

3.2.1 DNMT inhibitors

During preparation of genetic information in the S phase of the cell cycle, replication machinery is responsible for DNA replication, and DNMT functions duplicate methylation status by adding methyl groups to the DNA accordingly (**Figure 6**). DNMT inhibitors, azacytidine and decitabine, prevent DNMT methylation. Azacytidine and decitabine are metabolized inside cells into 5-aza-2′-deoxycytidine-triphosphate. The difference between DNMT bounding to 5-aza-2′-deoxycytidine-triphosphate and DNMT bound to cytosine is used to inhibit DNMT. As illustrated in **Figure 7**, DNMT reversibly binds with cytosine, which allows DNMT to be released from DNA through beta-elimination once methylation is completed. DNMT binding to 5-aza-2′-deoxycytidine-triphosphate establishes a covalent bond preventing beta-elimination; therefore, DNMT remains bond to the DNA. Subsequently, the error triggers DNA damage signaling and the trapped DNMT is degraded. As a result, methylation markers get lost during DNA replication [78]. Demethylated DNA allows for an open chromatin structure to be accessed by transcription factors induce by chemotherapeutic drugs such as glucocorticoids.

Single-agent study conducted by Khaldoun Al-Romaih's group showed that decitabine therapy had a cytotoxic effect mediated by the removal of hypomethylation of the CpG position both in vivo and in vitro. The cells treated with decitabine showed significant cell death in vitro, and six pro-apoptotic genes (GADD45A, HSPA9B, PAWR, PDCD5, NFKBIA, and TNFAIP3) were induced to ≥ twofold in vivo [79]. Combination therapy trials revealed the value of DNMT inhibition in addition to current therapeutic regimens. In one clinical trial in refractory ALL patients, decitabine combined with hyper-CVAD (fractionated cyclophosphamide, vincristine, doxorubicin, and dexamethasone alternating with high-dose methotrexate and cytarabine) was able to achieve complete remission in patients that did

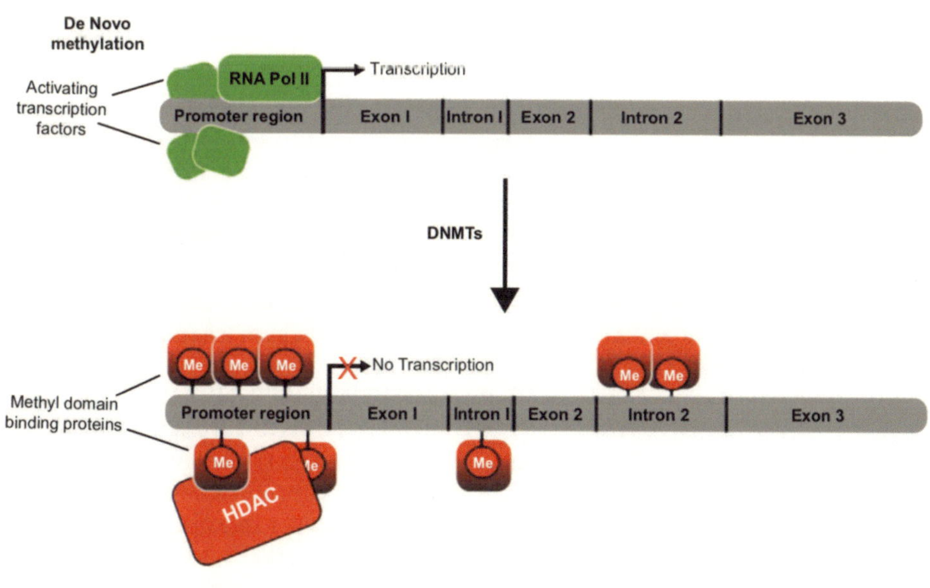

Figure 6.
Effect of epigenetic modification on gene expression. Activation of gene transcription needs transcription factor binding to the promoter region of the gene. Without DNA methylation, transcription factors and RNA polymerase II (RNA pol II) can bind to DNA segments; however, when methyl group is added to the DNA by DNA methyltransferase (DNMT), the methylation not only impedes the binding of transcription factors to DNA but also recruits histone deacetylase (HDAC) causing chromatin structure to become compacted, which places spatial limitation for transcription factor binding [83].

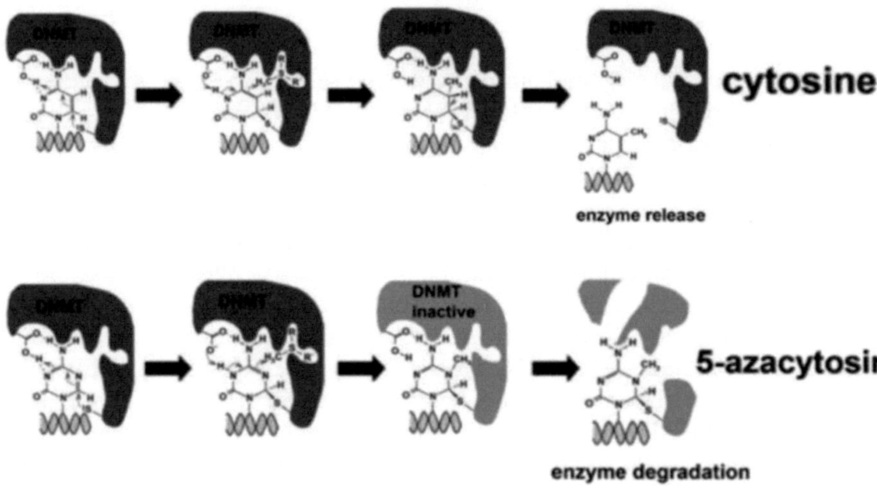

Figure 7.
Reversible binding of cytosine with DNMT in DNA methylation process versus irreversible binding of 5-azacytosine with DNMT when leukemia cells were treated with azacytidine, which leads to degradation of DNMT and subsequent loss of methylation. Adapted from Stresemann and Lyko, 2008 [78].

not respond to hyper-CVAD treatment alone. Patient DNA analysis confirmed that the hypomethylation status in the combination treatment group was the reason for reversal of resistance [80]. A number of other clinical studies provided similar results, showing synergistic effects between hypomethylating agents and several chemotherapy agents. Agents such as prednisolone, etoposides, doxorubicin, and cytarabine were shown to increase chemosensitivity in leukemia cells [81–84]. Although promising not all experimental groups responded, indicating the need for further research into the complex network of interactions.

3.2.2 HDAC inhibitors

An open chromatin structure also relies on the relatively loose interactions between DNA and histone proteins. The addition of an acetyl groups to the lysine amino acids on histone proteins by histone acetyltransferases (HATs) reduces the positive charges on the histone proteins. DNA, negatively charged, is therefore less attracted to these now less positive histones, thus less tightly bound and easier for transcription factors to access [83]. Conversely, the removal of acetylation by histone deacetylase (HDAC) forms condensed heterochromatin and silences critical apoptosis gene transcriptions. HDAC inhibitors prevent this form of gene silencing and are used alongside standard chemotherapy to promote pro-apoptotic pathways.

HDAC enzyme family consists of Class I (HDAC1, HDAC2, HDAC3, HDAC8), Class II (HDAC4, HDAC5, HDAC6, HDAC7, HDAC9, HDAC10), Class III (SIRT1, SIRT2, SIRT3, SIRT4, SIRT5, SIRT6, and SIRT7), and Class IV (HDAC11). HDAC inhibitors are designed as either selective inhibitors or pan-inhibitors (against all types of HDAC). Evidence that some HDACs play a stronger role in cancer development and patient prognosis than others makes specific HDAC inhibitors more appealing for clinical use. A study of 94 pediatric ALL patients showed differential HDAC expressions between the T-ALL and B-ALL subtypes. For T-ALL, HDAC1 and HDAC4 showed a higher expression than in B-ALL. T-ALL patients with HDAC3 expression above the cohort median also displayed a significantly higher 5-year event-free survival (EFS). In B-ALL, HDAC5 had higher expression than in T-ALL. In both T-cell and B-cell ALL, HDAC7 and HADC9 expression levels higher than the cohort median were associated with a lower 5-year EFS [85]. These trends suggest that Class II HDACs are associated with poorer prognosis; hence, a specific inhibition of this class of HDACs is important.

3.2.3 Bromodomain inhibitors

Bromodomains (BRDs) are epigenetic readers which selectively bind to acetylate lysine of histones tails, regulating gene expression [86]. Bromodomain-containing proteins that target genes are primarily cell cycle M/G1 genes in mitotic chromatin (expressed at the end or immediately after mitosis); late-phase genes were not found to be BRD4 bound. M/G1 gene expression during telophase coincides with histone H3 and H4 acetylation in those genes. BRD binding to M/G1 genes was associated with recruitment of positive transcription elongation factor b (P-TEFb), resulting in translational memory in the daughter cells [87]. BRD binds to MYC and activates enhancer-binding protein 4 (AP4) promoters. AP4 is a key mediator of mitogenicity for proto-oncogene MYC [88]. Upon AP4 activation by MYC, repressing cell cycle arrests gene *P21* [88].

JQ1 is a BRD inhibitor which acts on the MYC-AP4 axis [89]. Direct inhibition by JQ1 of BRD binding to the MYC and AP4 promoters indirectly results in cell cycle arrest as a *P21*-induced response to DNA damage P53 or TGFb/Smad signaling pathways [90].

3.3 Epigenetic drugs in chemotherapy

Epigenetic drugs are useful in combination with cytotoxic drugs, due to their ability to allow for access to pro-apoptotic pathways, otherwise blocked by epigenetic silencing. In a subset of leukemia patients, resistance to cytotoxic drugs such as glucocorticoids and methotrexate is a result of inaction of pro-apoptotic genes. Theoretically, applying epigenetic drugs such as those mentioned above should remove the epigenetic modification such that pro-apoptotic genes may go from repression to promotion.

3.3.1 Epigenetic drugs to treat glucocorticoid resistance

Chromatin conformation and gene expression studies at the glucocorticoid-induced pro-apoptotic *BIM* gene in drug-sensitive versus resisted lymphoid cells indicated that glucocorticoid resistance in ALL patients may be due to epigenetic modifications.

3.3.2 DNMT inhibitors

Studies showed closed DNMT catalyzed chromatin structure caused by DNA methylation impedes the transcription of *BIM*; lymphocyte-specific open chromatin structure determines *BIM* expression. Therefore, modifying chromatin structure would allow for *BIM* expression. Common cytosine analog hypomethylating drugs, decitabine or azacytidine, used in ALL act by inhibiting DNMT activity thus reactivate silenced genes. Once metabolized inside cells into 5-aza-2′-deoxycytidine-triphosphate, cytosine substrates on DNA replication machinery are replaced by the drug analog. These DNMT inhibitors have been proven to work synergistically with glucocorticoids in glucocorticoid-resistant ALLs, increasing the overall effectiveness of the therapeutic regimens [84].

3.3.3 HDAC inhibitors

Suberoylanilide hydroxamic acid (SAHA; Vorinostat) is an HDAC inhibitor shown to work synergistically with different chemotherapies. Glucocorticoid-resistant ALL cases were associated to a correlation between histone H3K9 deacetylation and pro-apoptotic gene, *BIM*, repression [91, 92]. SAHA acts to increase acetylation at H3K9 for *BIM* expression. Another chemocytotoxic pathway involves FPGS conversion of methotrexate to a cytotoxic product responsible for apoptosis, MTX-PGs. HDAC1 represses *FPGS* via epigenetically silencing. The combination of SAHA with methotrexate was shown to increase *FPGS* expression by two- to fivefolds, thus increasing cytotoxic activity [93].

3.4 Combination therapy

Combination therapy aims to bring synergistic effects by targeting both cell death pathway (chemotherapy, e.g., glucocorticoids) and access to this pathway (epigenetic drug). Of the clinical trials underway, the use of relatively high doses of 5-azacitidine (150 mg/m^2 as a continuous infusion daily × 5 days) is combined with cytarabine in patients relapsed from cytarabine alone. It was hypothesized that treatment with 5-azacitidine could induce expression of deoxycytidine kinase. Two out of the 17 patients achieved complete responses (CR). In another study, decitabine was combined with either amsacrine or idarubicin in patients with acute leukemia. CR was achieved in 36% (23 out 63) of patients, with a median disease-free survival of 8 months [82].

Using a hypomethylating agent such as decitabine, glucocorticoids in resistant ALL patients had the potential to expose the pro-apoptotic gene *BIM*, making it available for GR binding and subsequent transcription; thus reversing patient glucocorticoid resistance [5]. This should especially increase the rate of CR among the patients with glucocorticoid-resistant ALL and prolong event-free survival as suggested in preclinical trial model.

4. Conclusion

Knowledge of gene regulation has deepened the understanding of cellular mechanisms and disease development. In leukemia, genomic and epigenomic landscapes together provide crucial disease mechanism of pathogenicity and drug resistance [94–96]. Epigenetics is the driver of life and diversity of different organisms, and equally able to dysregulate cells and cause diseases such as leukemia. Hematopoiesis is a tightly controlled process essential for life, therefore, unless appropriately regulated, susceptible to regulatory errors as oncogenic drivers alongside mutations. Lineage-specific landscapes have been shown to be involved in hematopoiesis and leukemia evolution [51], providing a backbone for understanding targetable and non-targetable sites within different leukemic subtypes.

Studying a level of cell dysfunction preceding DNA mutations has allowed for understanding into pathogenesis and drug resistance which could not be correlated to DNA sequencing. Understanding resistance to chemotherapies, lowering patient prognosis, has been enlightened in epigenetic studies. For example, actions of glucocorticoids are cell type-specific and can be used in lymphocyte-specific leukemia cells to induce cell death [66, 67]. Analysis between genome-wide lymphocyte-specific open chromatin domains (LSOs) and integrated LSOs with glucocorticoid-induced RNA transcription and chromatin modulation in ALL was performed to causes glucocorticoid resistance beyond gene mutations [5]. LSOs critical for glucocorticoid-induced apoptosis were identified as well as structural protein CTCF binding in this region. These findings showed that upon GR binding to the LSO and CTCF binding, DNA would loop at the pro-apoptotic *BIM* gene and could be expressed. Crucially, DNA methylation (closed chromatin structure) was present in glucocorticoid-resistant ALL and nonlymphoid cell types, preventing DNA looping and *BIM* expression.

Understanding the importance of chromatin accessibility has allowed for identification of glucocorticoid sensitivity in cells and provides promising drug response predictions. Furthermore, development of epigenetic drugs that may modify chromatin to be accessible is currently being investigated. This would allow for more effective drug treatments to disrupt the oncogenesis driven via dysregulated pathways.

Author details

Bingzhi He†, Julia Cathryn Hlavka-Zhang†, Richard B. Lock and Duohui Jing*
Children's Cancer Institute, Lowy Cancer Research Centre, UNSW, Sydney, NSW, Australia

*Address all correspondence to: djing@ccia.unsw.edu.au

†Both authors contributed equally to this work

References

[1] Amin V et al. Epigenomic footprints across 111 reference epigenomes reveal tissue-specific epigenetic regulation of lincRNAs. Nature Communications. 2015;**6**:6370

[2] Ziller MJ et al. Dissecting neural differentiation regulatory networks through epigenetic footprinting. Nature. 2015;**518**(7539):355-359

[3] Dixon JR et al. Chromatin architecture reorganization during stem cell differentiation. Nature. 2015;**518**(7539):331-336

[4] De Jager PL et al. Alzheimer's disease: Early alterations in brain DNA methylation at ANK1, BIN1, RHBDF2 and other loci. Nature Neuroscience. 2014;**17**(9):1156-1163

[5] Jing D et al. Lymphocyte-specific chromatin accessibility pre-determines glucocorticoid resistance in acute lymphoblastic leukemia. Cancer Cell. 2018;**34**(6):906-921 e8

[6] Alvarez-Errico D et al. Epigenetic control of myeloid cell differentiation, identity and function. Nature Reviews. Immunology. 2015;**15**(1):7-17

[7] Luger K, Dechassa ML, Tremethick DJ. New insights into nucleosome and chromatin structure: An ordered state or a disordered affair? Nature Reviews. Molecular Cell Biology. 2012;**13**(7):436-447

[8] John S et al. Chromatin accessibility pre-determines glucocorticoid receptor binding patterns. Nature Genetics. 2011;**43**(3):264-268

[9] Margueron R, Reinberg D. Chromatin structure and the inheritance of epigenetic information. Nature Reviews. Genetics. 2010;**11**(4):285-296

[10] Shlyueva D, Stampfel G, Stark A. Transcriptional enhancers: From properties to genome-wide predictions. Nature Reviews. Genetics. 2014;**15**(4):272-286

[11] Aranda S, Mas G, Di Croce L. Regulation of gene transcription by polycomb proteins. Science Advances. 2015;**1**(11):e1500737

[12] Wiemels J. Perspectives on the causes of childhood leukemia. Chemico-Biological Interactions. 2012;**196**(3):59-67

[13] Gilham C et al. Day care in infancy and risk of childhood acute lymphoblastic leukaemia: Findings from UK case-control study. BMJ. 2005;**330**(7503):1294

[14] Mullighan CG. The genomic landscape of acute lymphoblastic leukemia in children and young adults. Hematology. American Society of Hematology. Education Program. 2014;**2014**(1):174-180

[15] Mullighan CG. Genomic characterization of childhood acute lymphoblastic leukemia. Seminars in Hematology. 2013;**50**(4):314-324

[16] Dang J et al. PAX5 is a tumor suppressor in mouse mutagenesis models of acute lymphoblastic leukemia. Blood. 2015;**125**(23):3609-3617

[17] Pui CH, Robison LL, Look AT. Acute lymphoblastic leukaemia. Lancet. 2008;**371**(9617):1030-1043

[18] Roberts KG, Mullighan CG. Genomics in acute lymphoblastic leukaemia: Insights and treatment implications. Nature Reviews. Clinical Oncology. 2015;**12**(6):344-357

[19] Bercovich D et al. Mutations of JAK2 in acute lymphoblastic leukaemias

associated with down's syndrome. Lancet. 2008;**372**(9648):1484-1492

[20] Levine RL. Inherited susceptibility to pediatric acute lymphoblastic leukemia. Nature Genetics. 2009;**41**(9):957-958

[21] Zuckerman T, Rowe JM. Pathogenesis and prognostication in acute lymphoblastic leukemia. F1000Prime Reports. 2014;**6**:59

[22] Hunger SP, Mullighan CG. Acute lymphoblastic leukemia in children. The New England Journal of Medicine. 2015;**373**(16):1541-1552

[23] Swaminathan S et al. Mechanisms of clonal evolution in childhood acute lymphoblastic leukemia. Nature Immunology. 2015;**16**(7):766-774

[24] Ford AM et al. Fetal origins of the TEL-AML1 fusion gene in identical twins with leukemia. Proceedings of the National Academy of Sciences of the United States of America. 1998;**95**(8):4584-4588

[25] Wasserman R et al. Predominance of fetal type DJH joining in young children with B precursor lymphoblastic leukemia as evidence for an in utero transforming event. The Journal of Experimental Medicine. 1992;**176**(6):1577-1581

[26] Francis SS et al. Mode of delivery and risk of childhood leukemia. Cancer Epidemiology, Biomarkers & Prevention. 2014;**23**(5):876-881

[27] Copley MR, Eaves CJ. Developmental changes in hematopoietic stem cell properties. Experimental and Molecular Medicine. 2013;**45**:e55

[28] Jing D et al. Opposing regulation of BIM and BCL2 controls glucocorticoid-induced apoptosis of pediatric acute lymphoblastic leukemia cells. Blood. 2015;**125**(2):273-283

[29] Crawford GE et al. Genome-wide mapping of DNase hypersensitive sites using massively parallel signature sequencing (MPSS). Genome Research. 2006;**16**(1):123-131

[30] Wiench M et al. DNA methylation status predicts cell type-specific enhancer activity. The EMBO Journal. 2011;**30**(15):3028-3039

[31] Schindler JW et al. TEL-AML1 corrupts hematopoietic stem cells to persist in the bone marrow and initiate leukemia. Cell Stem Cell. 2009;**5**(1):43-53

[32] Zelent A, Greaves M, Enver T. Role of the TEL-AML1 fusion gene in the molecular pathogenesis of childhood acute lymphoblastic leukaemia. Oncogene. 2004;**23**(24):4275-4283

[33] Armstrong SA, Look AT. Molecular genetics of acute lymphoblastic leukemia. Journal of Clinical Oncology. 2005;**23**(26):6306-6315

[34] Di Cello F et al. Inactivation of the Cdkn2a locus cooperates with HMGA1 to drive T-cell leukemogenesis. Leukemia & Lymphoma. 2013;**54**(8):1762-1768

[35] Pui CH, Relling MV, Downing JR. Acute lymphoblastic leukemia. The New England Journal of Medicine. 2004;**350**(15):1535-1548

[36] Mullighan CG et al. Genome-wide analysis of genetic alterations in acute lymphoblastic leukaemia. Nature. 2007;**446**(7137):758-764

[37] Speck NA, Gilliland DG. Core-binding factors in haematopoiesis and leukaemia. Nature Reviews Cancer. 2002;**2**(7):502-513

[38] Torpy JM, Lynm C, Glass RM. JAMA patient page. Acute lymphoblastic leukemia. JAMA. 2009;**301**(4):452

[39] Goulding NJ, Flower RJ. Glucocorticoids, Milestones in drug therapy. Basel, Switzerland: Boston: Birkhäuser Verlag; 2001. p. 205

[40] Dalakas MC. Inflammatory muscle diseases. The New England Journal of Medicine. 2015;**372**(18):1734-1747

[41] Nair P et al. Oral glucocorticoid-sparing effect of benralizumab in severe asthma. The New England Journal of Medicine. 2017;**376**(25):2448-2458

[42] Inaba H, Pui CH. Glucocorticoid use in acute lymphoblastic leukaemia. The Lancet Oncology. 2010;**11**(11):1096-1106

[43] Kim IK et al. Glucocorticoid-induced tumor necrosis factor receptor-related protein co-stimulation facilitates tumor regression by inducing IL-9-producing helper T cells. Nature Medicine. 2015;**21**(9):1010-1017

[44] Palumbo A et al. Daratumumab, bortezomib, and dexamethasone for multiple myeloma. The New England Journal of Medicine. 2016;**375**(8):754-766

[45] Pui CH, Evans WE. A 50-year journey to cure childhood acute lymphoblastic leukemia. Seminars in Hematology. 2013;**50**(3):185-196

[46] Klumper E et al. In vitro cellular drug resistance in children with relapsed/refractory acute lymphoblastic leukemia. Blood. 1995;**86**(10):3861-3868

[47] Howard SC et al. Urolithiasis in pediatric patients with acute lymphoblastic leukemia. Leukemia. 2003;**17**(3):541-546

[48] Australian Institute of Health and Welfare. A Picture of Australia's Children 2012. Canberra: Australian Institute of Health and Welfare; 2012

[49] Guenther MG et al. A chromatin landmark and transcription initiation at most promoters in human cells. Cell. 2007;**130**(1):77-88

[50] Li G et al. Extensive promoter-centered chromatin interactions provide a topological basis for transcription regulation. Cell. 2012;**148**(1-2):84-98

[51] Corces MR et al. Lineage-specific and single-cell chromatin accessibility charts human hematopoiesis and leukemia evolution. Nature Genetics. 2016;**48**(10):1193-1203

[52] Hnisz D, Day DS, Young RA. Insulated neighborhoods: Structural and functional units of mammalian gene control. Cell. 2016;**167**(5):1188-1200

[53] Thurman RE et al. The accessible chromatin landscape of the human genome. Nature. 2012;**489**(7414):75-82

[54] Perera D et al. Differential DNA repair underlies mutation hotspots at active promoters in cancer genomes. Nature. 2016;**532**(7598):259-263

[55] Greenstein S et al. Mechanisms of glucocorticoid-mediated apoptosis in hematological malignancies. Clinical Cancer Research. 2002;**8**(6):1681-1694

[56] Watson LC et al. The glucocorticoid receptor dimer interface allosterically transmits sequence-specific DNA signals. Nature Structural & Molecular Biology. 2013;**20**(7):876-883

[57] John S et al. Interaction of the glucocorticoid receptor with the chromatin landscape. Molecular Cell. 2008;**29**(5):611-624

[58] Paakinaho V et al. Glucocorticoid receptor activates poised FKBP51 locus through long-distance interactions. Molecular Endocrinology. 2010;**24**(3):511-525

[59] Vockley CM et al. Direct GR binding sites potentiate clusters of TF

binding across the human genome. Cell. 2016;**166**(5):1269-1281 e19

[60] Guo B et al. Glucocorticoid hormone-induced chromatin remodeling enhances human hematopoietic stem cell homing and engraftment. Nature Medicine. 2017;**23**(4):424-428

[61] Swinstead EE et al. Steroid receptors reprogram FoxA1 occupancy through dynamic chromatin transitions. Cell. 2016;**165**(3):593-605

[62] Love MI et al. Role of the chromatin landscape and sequence in determining cell type-specific genomic glucocorticoid receptor binding and gene regulation. Nucleic Acids Research. 2017;**45**(4):1805-1819

[63] Gross KL, Lu NZ, Cidlowski JA. Molecular mechanisms regulating glucocorticoid sensitivity and resistance. Molecular and Cellular Endocrinology. 2009;**300**(1-2):7-16

[64] Wasim M et al. PLZF/ZBTB16, a glucocorticoid response gene in acute lymphoblastic leukemia, interferes with glucocorticoid-induced apoptosis. The Journal of Steroid Biochemistry and Molecular Biology. 2010;**120**(4-5):218-227

[65] Klein K et al. Glucocorticoid-induced proliferation in untreated pediatric acute myeloid leukemic blasts. Pediatric Blood & Cancer. 2016;**63**(8):1457-1460

[66] Gruver-Yates AL, Cidlowski JA. Tissue-specific actions of glucocorticoids on apoptosis: A double-edged sword. Cell. 2013;**2**(2):202-223

[67] Cain DW, Cidlowski JA. Immune regulation by glucocorticoids. Nature Reviews. Immunology. 2017;**17**(4):233-247

[68] Ploner C et al. Glucocorticoid-induced apoptosis and glucocorticoid resistance in acute lymphoblastic leukemia. The Journal of Steroid Biochemistry and Molecular Biology. 2005;**93**(2-5):153-160

[69] Schmidt S et al. Glucocorticoid resistance in two key models of acute lymphoblastic leukemia occurs at the level of the glucocorticoid receptor. The FASEB Journal. 2006;**20**(14):2600-2602

[70] Piovan E et al. Direct reversal of glucocorticoid resistance by AKT inhibition in acute lymphoblastic leukemia. Cancer Cell. 2013;**24**(6):766-776

[71] van Galen JC et al. BTG1 regulates glucocorticoid receptor autoinduction in acute lymphoblastic leukemia. Blood. 2010;**115**(23):4810-4819

[72] Bachmann PS et al. Divergent mechanisms of glucocorticoid resistance in experimental models of pediatric acute lymphoblastic leukemia. Cancer Research. 2007;**67**(9):4482-4490

[73] Jones CL et al. MAPK signaling cascades mediate distinct glucocorticoid resistance mechanisms in pediatric leukemia. Blood. 2015;**126**(19):2202-2212

[74] Serafin V et al. Glucocorticoid resistance is reverted by LCK inhibition in pediatric T-cell acute lymphoblastic leukemia. Blood. 2017;**130**(25):2750-2761

[75] Nagao K, Iwai Y, Miyashita T. RCAN1 is an important mediator of glucocorticoid-induced apoptosis in human leukemic cells. PLoS One. 2012;**7**(11):e49926

[76] Cialfi S et al. Glucocorticoid sensitivity of T-cell lymphoblastic leukemia/lymphoma is associated with glucocorticoid receptor-mediated inhibition of Notch1 expression. Leukemia. 2013;**27**(2):485-488

[77] Falkenberg KJ, Johnstone RW. Histone deacetylases and their inhibitors in cancer, neurological diseases and immune disorders. Nature Reviews. Drug Discovery. 2014;**13**(9):673-691

[78] Stresemann C, Lyko F. Modes of action of the DNA methyltransferase inhibitors azacytidine and decitabine. International Journal of Cancer. 2008;**123**(1):8-13

[79] Al-Romaih K et al. Modulation by decitabine of gene expression and growth of osteosarcoma U2OS cells in vitro and in xenografts: Identification of apoptotic genes as targets for demethylation. Cancer Cell International. 2007;**7**:14

[80] Benton CB et al. Safety and clinical activity of 5-aza-2′-deoxycytidine (decitabine) with or without hyper-CVAD in relapsed/refractory acute lymphocytic leukaemia. British Journal of Haematology. 2014;**167**(3):356-365

[81] Garcia-Manero G et al. DNA methylation of multiple promoter-associated CpG islands in adult acute lymphocytic leukemia. Clinical Cancer Research. 2002;**8**(7):2217-2224

[82] Garcia-Manero G et al. Epigenetics of acute lymphocytic leukemia. Seminars in Hematology. 2009;**46**(1):24-32. DOI: 10.1053/j.seminhematol.2008.09.008

[83] Heerboth S et al. Use of epigenetic drugs in disease: An overview. Genetics & Epigenetics. 2014;**6**:9-19

[84] Lu BY et al. Decitabine enhances chemosensitivity of early T-cell precursor-acute lymphoblastic leukemia cell lines and patient-derived samples. Leukemia & Lymphoma. 2016;**57**(8):1938-1941

[85] Moreno DA et al. Research paper: Differential expression of HDAC3, HDAC7 and HDAC9 is associated with prognosis and survival in childhood acute lymphoblastic leukaemia. British Journal of Haematology. 2010;**150**(6):665-673

[86] Fujisawa T, Filippakopoulos P. Functions of bromodomain-containing proteins and their roles in homeostasis and cancer. Nature Reviews Molecular Cell Biology. 2017;**18**:246

[87] Dey A et al. Brd4 marks select genes on mitotic chromatin and directs postmitotic transcription. Molecular Biology of the Cell. 2009;**20**(23):4899-4909

[88] Choi SK et al. JQ1, an inhibitor of the epigenetic reader BRD4, suppresses the bidirectional MYC-AP4 axis via multiple mechanisms. Oncology Reports. 2016;**35**(2):1186

[89] Delmore JE et al. BET bromodomain inhibition as a therapeutic strategy to target c-Myc. Cell. 2011;**146**(6):904-917

[90] Jung P, Hermeking H. The c-MYC-AP4-p21 cascade. Cell Cycle. 2009;**8**(7):982-989

[91] Lock RB et al. Epigenetic silencing of the pro-apoptotic Bim gene in glucocorticoid poor-responsive pediatric acute lymphoblastic leukemia, and its reversal by histone deacetylase inhibition. Blood. 2009;**114**(22):939

[92] Zhang C et al. Histone acetylation: Novel target for the treatment of acute lymphoblastic leukemia. Clinical Epigenetics. 2015;**7**:117

[93] Leclerc GJ et al. Histone deacetylase inhibitors induce FPGS mRNA expression and intracellular accumulation of long-chain methotrexate polyglutamates in childhood acute lymphoblastic leukemia: Implications for combination therapy. Leukemia. 2010;**24**(3):552

[94] Cancer Genome Atlas Research, N et al. Genomic and epigenomic landscapes of adult de novo acute myeloid leukemia. The New England Journal of Medicine. 2013;**368**(22):2059-2074

[95] Hnisz D et al. Activation of proto-oncogenes by disruption of chromosome neighborhoods. Science. 2016;**351**(6280):1454-1458

[96] Iacobucci I, Mullighan CG. Genetic basis of acute lymphoblastic leukemia. Journal of Clinical Oncology. 2017;**35**(9):975-983

[97] Australian Institute of Health and Welfare (AIHW). Australian Cancer Incidence and Mortality (ACIM) Books: Acute Lymphoblastic Leukaemia. Canberra: AIHW; 2014

Section 3

Germ Line Mutations Associated Leukemia

Chapter 3

Familial Leukemia Associated with Thrombocytopenia

Jakub Trizuljak and Michael Doubek

Abstract

Familial predisposition to leukemia has been known for decades. In some families, this condition is also associated with thrombocytopenia and history of bleeding. Germline mutations in the RUNX1 gene have been proven to cause familial platelet disorder with predisposition to myeloid malignancies (FDPMM). The disease typically presents with mild-to-moderate thrombocytopenia with normal-size platelets, functional platelet defects leading to prolonged bleeding, and an increased risk to develop myelodysplastic syndrome (MDS), acute myeloid leukemia (AML), or T-cell acute lymphoblastic leukemia (T-ALL). In recent years, molecular defects in other genes, such as ANKRD26 and ETV6, have been associated with thrombocytopenia and susceptibility to hematological malignancy as well. In our chapter, we will present a review of up-to-date knowledge on this topic along with several case studies demonstrating the diagnostic process and management of the affected families.

Keywords: AML, familial, RUNX1, ANKRD26, ETV6

1. Introduction

Familial leukemia (e.g., repeated occurrence of hematologic neoplasia in families more often than is expected by chance alone) has been a topic of interest for decades. Almost a hundred years ago, connections between inherited forms of myelodysplastic syndrome (MDS) and myeloid and lymphoid leukemia were established with several constitutional disorders in childhood, such as Fanconi anemia [1]. Since then, a number of additional inherited bone marrow failure syndromes and inherited conditions with predisposition to leukemia were discovered. Repeated occurrence of similar phenotypes, high clinical penetrance for hematologic disorders, and often consanguineous inheritance made identification of the respective genetic causes easier. These conditions are caused by germline mutations (genetic changes which can be carried on to next generations) in genes playing an important role in the development and maintenance of hematopoietic system. Collective effort of many researchers in the past has improved the knowledge about risk for MDS/leukemia, as well as the natural history and clinical outcomes of affected patients [2].

Some of these syndromes present with a distinctive hematological phenotype—thrombocytopenia. Until the end of the last century, only a few forms of inherited thrombocytopenia were known, all of which were extremely rare. Since then, the knowledge of thrombocytopenia has improved, and we presently know at least 26 disorders caused by mutations in 30 genes [3]. It also became quite apparent that in

Myeloid neoplasm classification	Genes involved	Recurrently mutated in sporadic AML, largely initiating or secondary event
Myeloid neoplasma without a preexisting disorder or organ dysfunction	*CEBPA*	Yes, secondary
	DDX41	No
Myeloid neoplasms and preexisting platelet disorders	*RUNX1*	Yes, secondary
	ANKRD26	No
	ETV6	Yes, secondary
Myeloid neoplasm and other organ dysfunction		
Germ line *GATA2* mutation	*GATA2*	Yes, secondary
BM failure syndromes*	*Multiple*	No
Telomere biology disorders	*TERT, TERK*	No
JMML associated with neurofibromatosis, Noonan syndrome or Noonan syndrome-like disorders, Down syndrome	*NF1, PTPN11, CBL, KRAS*	Yes, secondary

** Includes Fanconi anemia (FANCA, FANCB, FANCC, FANCD1 (BRCA1), FANCD2, FANCE, FANCF, FANCG, FANCI, FANCJ (BRIP1), FANCL, FANCM, FANCN (PALB2), FANCO (RAD51C), FANCP (SLX4), FANCQ (ERCC4), FANCR (RAD51), FANCS (BRCA1), FANCT (UBE2T), FANCU, (XRCC2), FANCV (MAD2L2/REV7) and FANCW (RFWD3)), dyskeratosis congenita (DKC1, TERC, TERT, TIN2, NOP10, NHP2), Schwachman-Diamond syndrome (SBDS), Diamond Blackfan anemia (RPS19, RPS24, RPs17, RPL5, RPL11, RPL35A, RPS7, RPS10, RPs26, GATA1), congenital amegakaryocytic thrombocytopenia (MPL), and severe congenital neutropenia (ELA2, GFI1, HAX1).*

Figure 1.
Myeloid malignancies with germline predisposition. The 2016 revision to the World Health Organization classification of myeloid neoplasms and acute leukemia [4].

some families, there is a connection between thrombocytopenia and additional risk of hematological malignancy. Thanks to availability of next-generation sequencing (NGS) technologies, genes associated with hereditary thrombocytopenia and risk of leukemic transformation were successfully identified, notably RUNX1, ETV6, and ANKRD26. These new hereditary syndromes were included in the 2016 revision of World Health Organization (WHO) classification of myeloid neoplasms and acute leukemia [4] **(Figure 1)**.

2. *RUNX1* deficiency (familial platelet disorder with predisposition to myeloid malignancies (FPDMM))

RUNT-related transcription factor 1 (RUNX1) is a master regulator of hematopoiesis [5]. It is involved in the most frequent chromosome translocations in leukemia (i.e., t (12;21)/*RUNX1/ETV6*, t(8;21)/*RUNX1/RUNX1T1*, and t(3;21)/*RUNX1/EVI1*) [6]. Moreover, somatic *RUNX1* mutations have been identified as recurrent abnormalities in myelodysplastic syndromes (MDS) and acute myeloid leukemia (AML) [7].

For the first time, germline *RUNX1* mutations were described in 1999 [8]. Individuals carrying germline *RUNX1* mutation may develop familial platelet disorder with predisposition to myeloid malignancies (FPDMM). Characteristic features include (1) thrombocytopenia, (2) functional platelet defects, and (3) an increased risk to develop MDS, AML, or acute T-lymphoblastic leukemia (T-ALL). There is a significant phenotypic heterogeneity. FPDMM (MIM601399) is inherited in an autosomal-dominant mode with incomplete penetrance and variable expressivity [5, 6].

2.1 Diagnostic criteria to identify at-risk individuals

Diagnosis of FDPMM in patients with leukemia carries important clinical implications for the patient but also for her/his family. Recognition of clinical features pointing to this genetic predisposition is crucial. The most important feature is persistent thrombocytopenia or aspirin-like platelet disorder. Pedigree analysis can identify first- or second-degree relatives with higher occurrence of bleeding and hematological malignancies. The bleeding symptoms may be mild or not present. Onset of leukemia varies and spans from infant age to adulthood [9, 10]. In the case of family history of MDS, early-onset leukemia and/or a personal history of bleeding, immune deficiency, or dysmorphic features, genetic counseling is advised [11, 12]. Comprehensive evaluation involves a thorough review of individual's family and personal history, hematologic investigation, and personal risk assessment of likelihood of a hereditary predisposition within his/her family, and if necessary, genetic testing with NGS to determine the possibility of a germline mutation should be offered [13]. We provide an example of a familial case of FDPMM in **Figure 2** [14].

Predictive testing of healthy relatives is advised due to risk of bleeding and leukemia, even in infancy. In the case of individuals with leukemia, where allogenic stem cell transplantation from a HLA-matching sibling donor is the best possible treatment option, mutation screening should be a part of decision-making process, to prevent adverse outcomes after transplantation [15–17].

Due to the advance and widespread use of NGS technologies in diagnosis of myeloid neoplasia in recent years, many individuals at risk are being identified by screening large cohorts of patients. In particular, leukemias with homozygous RUNX1 mutations, biallelic RUNX1 mutations, and trisomy 21 indicate that the patients are likely candidates for FDPMM [18].

2.2 Platelet features

A personal or family history of thrombocytopenia and/or bleeding tendency may be an important pointer to diagnose FDPMM in patient with MDS, AML, or T-ALL. The platelet count is usually mild to moderate and, in some cases, low-normal and even normal. Platelet size is not affected—similar to ETV6- or ANKRD26-related thrombocytopenias, which are also characterized by normal-size platelets [19]. Thrombocytopenia is caused by abnormal megakaryocyte maturation and impaired proplatelet formation. Dysmegakaryopoiesis may be present in bone marrow smears even before leukemic transformation [20].

A functional defect of platelets is present in most, if not all, patients with RUNX1 germline mutations, leading to abnormal secretion and aggregation [21].

The bleeding diathesis is variable within and among families. As some carriers of RUNX1 have mild or none bleeding symptoms, the presence of mutation may go unnoticed, and genetic screening is necessary to determine mutational status.

2.3 Role of *RUNX1* in hematopoiesis

The finding of platelet abnormalities in patients with FDPMM has revealed the essential role of RUNX1 in the megakaryocytic lineage. RUNX1 works as a transcription factor at different stages of megakaryocyte development by regulating the expression of multiple factors relevant to platelet production and function. Reduced expression of RUNX1 target genes, including MPL proto-oncogene, thrombopoietin receptor (MPL), nonmuscle myosin IIA/myosin heavy chain 9 (MYH9) and its regulatory chain MLC2, arachidonate 12-lipoxygenase (ALOX12), and NFE2, has been shown to cause the defect in platelet number and function in FDPMM [22, 23]. What is more, increased levels

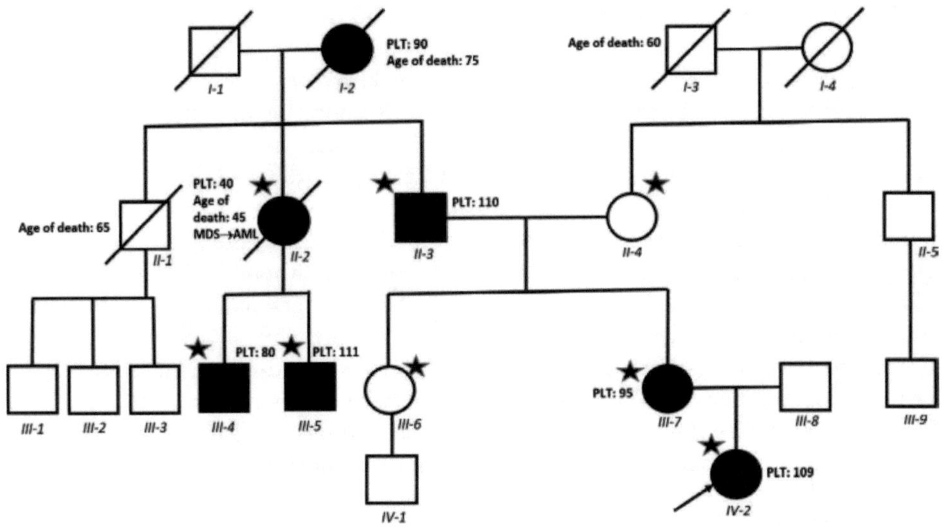

Figure 2.
*Pedigree of a family with thrombocytopenia and predisposition to myeloid malignancies. We identified a family with platelet disorder and predisposition to myeloid malignancies. Using exome sequencing of samples of eight family members, we identified a pathogenic frameshift variant c.866delG (p.Gly289Aspfs*22) in exon 8 of RUNX1 gene, resulting in a premature stop codon. The mutation occurs within the transactivation domain of RUNX1. One of the affected individuals developed myelodysplastic syndrome, which progressed to acute myelogenous leukemia. Platelet count (PLT) reported in ×109/L, samples analyzed by exome sequencing marked with an asterisk (*), age of death if known [14].*

of nonmuscle myosin IIB (MYH10), which is physiologically repressed by RUNX1, contribute to thrombocytopenia by blocking megakaryocyte polyploidization [24].

RUNX1 is a master regulator in hematopoietic differentiation. It plays a role in the first wave of hematopoiesis producing primitive erythroid cells and megakaryocytes. By enhanced expression of CEBPE, it negatively regulates myeloid progenitors and induces granulocytic differentiation. RUNX1 also regulates cell adhesion to the bone marrow niche [25]. After dimerizing with core-binding factor beta (CBFB), RUNX1 binds to promotor regions of several transcription factors like PU.1, regulating their expression. Binding to DNA and CBFB occurs in the highly conserved Runt homology domain (RHD) at the N-terminal region. Transactivation occurs at the C-terminal part of the molecule [26].

2.4 Phenotype/genotype correlation

Most RUNX1 mutations lie in the Runt homology domain region (RHD) [1]. Causative mutations are deleterious—most often frameshift, nonsense, or in/del mutations that result in premature protein truncation or nonsense-mediated decay of mRNA. Missense mutations may be present as well. In these cases, it may be hard to determine the pathogenicity of found variants. Here, segregation analyses and functional analyses are needed to confirm the effect of the variants for pathogenesis. Loss of function mutations in RHD, located in the N-terminal part of the protein, impairs normal RUNX1 function by hindering dimerization and DNA binding. These, as well as mutations in the 5′ regulatory region cause haploinsufficiency [27]. Missense mutations in RHD and nonsense and frameshift mutations in the C-terminal domain may lead to dominant-negative effects [10].

What is more, there are inherited structural rearrangements involving RUNX1: FDPMM can also be caused by small deletions involving a few base pairs or single exons of the gene and large deletions leading to loss of the complete coding regions.

Deletions of large parts of the long arm of chromosome 21 cause a contiguous gene with various clinical signs, e.g., facial dysmorphism, mental retardation, thrombocytopenia, and increased risk of myeloid malignancies. These large deletions can be reliably detected by array comparative genomic hybridization (CGH)/single-nucleotide polymorphism (SNP) arrays [11, 12].

There seems to be a higher risk of leukemic transformation in the case of dominant-negative mutations of RUNx1 as compared to loss-of-function mutations. Both types of alterations lead to thrombocytopenia phenotype, but only dominant-negative mutations enhance the proliferation rate and clonogenic potential [28]. In the case of haploinsufficiency, biallelic or second-hit mutations are needed to trigger the leukemic transformation.

Unfortunately, there is no clear phenotype/genotype correlation. Within one family, members carrying the same mutation may present with different clinical signs and severity of symptoms. Some carriers develop only mild thrombocytopenia, while others suffer from myeloid neoplasms [29].

2.5 Risk of malignancy and second-hit mutations in RUNX1 deficiency

The risk of malignant transformation into MDS or AML is estimated to be 30–40% [16]. Patients carrying dominant-negative RUNX1 mutations have a higher risk of malignant transformation. The spectrum of malignancies involves AML of various French-American-British subtypes and MDS (refractory anemia with excess blasts, chronic myelomonocytic leukemia and hypoplastic MDS with myelofibrosis). In some cases T-cell ALL has also been described. In the case of MDS/AML, age of onset is at an average of 33 years with a wide age range, while in T-cell ALL, it usually occurs at a younger age [13, 24].

During the course of the disease, the second allele may be inactivated, as expected for tumor suppressor genes according to two-hit hypothesis. Nowadays, there are no definitive answers to what triggers the malignant transformation in RUNX1 germline mutation carriers. However, clonal hematopoiesis may be present even in asymptomatic mutation carriers, preceding overt MDS/AML or FDPMM [30].

Carriers of RUNX1 germline mutations need additional genetic events to develop hematological neoplasm. Often, biallelic alterations of RUNX1 are found, due to secondary RUNx1 mutations or acquired trisomy 21 resulting in the duplication of the mutated allele [31]. RUNx1 mutations are associated with MLL partial tandem duplications, FLT3-ITD, IDH1/2, RAS mutations, and ETV6 rearrangements. These often occur in therapy-related AML [32]. Recently, malignant transformation was reported to be mediated by recurrent somatic mutations in CD25C gene in up to a half of a Japanese patient cohort with RUNX1-related myeloid neoplasia. Next-generation sequencing allows detection of additional mutations in known AML drivers, such as ASXL1, TET2, IDH1, CEBPD, RB1, MLI2, FLT3-ITD, WT1, and SRSF2 [33, 34].

2.6 Clinical management

Treatment of RUNX1-related AML or MDS follows standard protocols. If a disease-causing germline mutation is known in the family, it is important to prevent hematopoietic stem cell transplantation from a sibling or other relative.

In families with high-penetrance mutations, regular clinical examinations including differential blood count are advised. In case of suspicious clinical symptoms or cytopenias, bone marrow aspiration or biopsy with morphological, cytogenetic, and molecular genetic investigations should be discussed. Using new NGS technologies, it is possible to follow up clonal hematopoiesis [30].

2.7 Conclusion

RUNX1 deficiency is a myeloid malignancy predisposition syndrome with high clinical penetrance and variable expressivity of its phenotypic effects. An aspirin-like platelet and mild-to-moderate thrombocytopenia are present in most of the patients. The presence of possible RUNX1 germline mutations should be part of decision-making process in management of HSCT and donor choice in MDS/AML. Follow-up of asymptomatic mutation carriers is necessary.

3. ETV6-related thrombocytopenia with propensity to hematological malignancies

ETV6 was originally discovered in a leukemia-associated chromosomal translocation [35] and has subsequently been identified as a fusion partner in more than 30 chromosomal translocation oncogenes [36]. ETV6 is a transcriptional repressor that binds DNA via a C-terminal DNA-binding domain, highly conserved among ETS-family transcription factors [37]. The ETV6 N-terminal pointed (PNT) domain mediates self-association and frequently contributes to fusion proteins as the partner of tyrosine kinases [38]. Loss of ETV6 has firmly been implicated in the pathogenesis of ETV6-RUNX1(TEL-AML1)-associated childhood leukemia as there is invariably biallelic loss of ETV6 due to deletions of the second (nontranslocated) ETV6 allele [39].

More recently, genome-wide investigations have uncovered that ETV6 is subject to heterozygous mutations in hematologic malignancies, including myelodysplastic syndrome (MDS) [10, 11], acute myeloid leukemia (AML) [40], early T-cell precursor acute lymphoblastic leukemia (T-ALL) [41, 42], high-risk B-ALL [43], and diffuse large B-cell lymphoma (DLBCL) [44]. It remained unclear whether and how loss of ETV6 contributes to leukemogenesis.

Now a number of recent studies have expanded our knowledge. The initial report from Zhang et al. identified the link between heterozygous germline ETV6 mutation to dominantly inherited thrombocytopenia and predisposition to hematological malignancies [45]. Subsequent studies extended these findings to additional families with unique ETV6 germline mutations and predisposition to malignancy [46, 47]. With one exception, all of the germline mutations cluster within the highly conserved ETS domain. The only mutation outside the ETS domain, P214L, was repeatedly identified in family studies.

3.1 Diagnostic criteria to identify at-risk individuals

Diagnosis of ETV6-related thrombocytopenia is paramount due to clinical implications for the patient. The most important clinical feature is thrombocytopenia with normal-sized platelets. Sometimes, large mean corpuscular volume (MCV) of red blood cells is reported. In family history, individuals with occurrence of bleeding and hematological malignancies are identified. Bleeding symptoms are variable. No recurrent extra-hematologic abnormalities have been identified, though in some families, solid tumors may occur [45].

Genetic counseling, comprehensive evaluation of individual's family and personal history, hematologic investigation, personal risk assessment of likelihood of a hereditary predisposition within his/her family, and, if necessary, genetic testing with NGS are advised. In the case of a found mutation, predictive testing of healthy relatives is necessary to identify at-risk individuals [13]. We provide an example of a familial case of ETV6 deficiency in **Figure 3** [47]. In cases when allogenic hematopoietic stem-cell transplantation is considered in a patient with leukemia and ETV6 mutation, possible sibling donors must be tested to avoid the risk of relapse and transplant-related morbidity and mortality.

3.2 Platelet features

All affected pedigrees with ETV6 germline mutations have a highly penetrant autosomal-dominant pattern of thrombocytopenia. Severity of thrombocytopenia is highly variable. Many patients have mild thrombocytopenia with platelet counts ranging between 100 and 150 $\times 10^9$/L, while others had platelet counts $<50 \times 10^9$/L. Severe thrombocytopenia $<20 \times 10^9$/L is seen rarely in the absence of myelodysplastic syndrome [46]. Bleeding symptoms reported are generally mild including petechiae, ecchymoses, epistaxis, gum bleeding, easy bruising, and menorrhagia. Platelet size is generally normal, though macrothrombocytopenia may be seen in a subset of patients.

Hemoglobin is normal in most patients. Erythrocyte mean corpuscular volume (MCV) is generally normal or increased. Neutrophil counts are normal. Examination of bone marrow reveals frequent immature hypolobulated megakaryocytes, mild dyserythropoiesis, and mild hypolobulation and hypogranulation of myeloid cells [48].

3.3 Risk of malignancy

A substantial number of patients carrying ETV6 germline mutation develop hematological malignancies during their lifetime. The risk of leukemic transformation is estimated to be up to 25–40%; the age of onset is highly variable (8–82 years). The spectrum of malignancies involves acute lymphoblastic leukemia (ALL) and myeloid malignancies including MDS, AML, chronic myelomonocytic leukemia (CMML), myeloproliferative disorders (typically polycythemia vera), and multiple myeloma. Special attention was brought to relationship between germline ETV6 mutations and childhood ALL. Targeted sequencing of

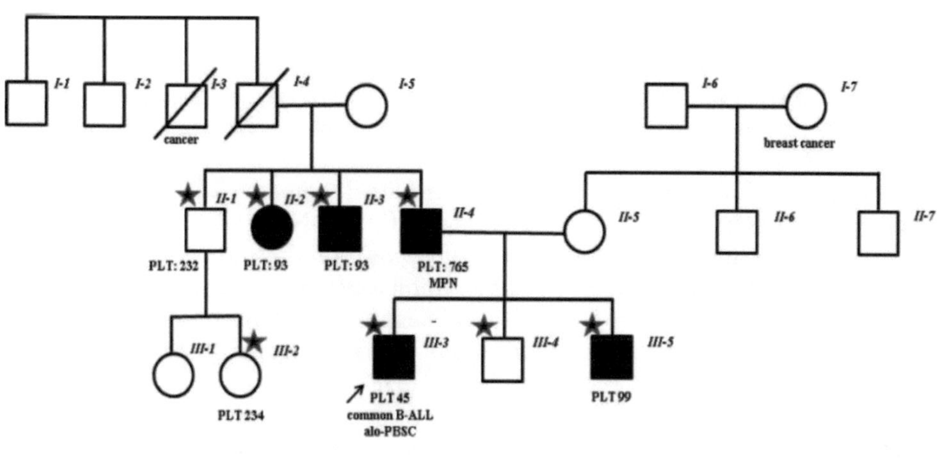

Figure 3.
Pedigree of a family with thrombocytopenia and occurrence of lymphoid and myeloid malignancies. We identified a family with autosomal dominant thrombocytopenia, high erythrocyte mean corpuscular volume (MCV), occurrence of B cell-precursor acute lymphoblastic leukemia (ALL) and myeloproliferative neoplasm (MPN). Whole-exome sequencing identified a heterozygous single-nucleotide change in ETV6 (ETS variant 6), c.1138T>A, encoding a p.Trp380Arg substitution in the C-terminal DNA-binding domain, segregating with thrombocytopenia and elevated MCV. The role of Trp380 is structural, being surrounded by hydrophobic residues in the domain hydrophobic core. Its substitution by an arginine will therefore severely destabilize the domain structure. Platelet count (PLT) reported in ×109/L, samples analyzed by exome sequencing marked with an asterisk [47].

a large cohort of childhood ALL patients revealed 31 leukemia-associated ETV6 exonic variants [49]. All variants in this study were absent in control population. About 48% of found variants were found in the ETS DNA-binding domain and were predicted to be deleterious. Children with ETV6 variants were older at diagnosis (median 10.2 years) than those without ETV6 variants (4.7 years). There was no association between ETV6 mutation status and early treatment response or risk of relapse.

In some families, a few sold tumors have been reported: colorectal carcinoma, breast cancer, renal cell carcinoma, and tumor of the central nervous system. Further investigation is needed to understand the role of ETV6 in solid tumors [45, 49, 50].

3.4 Mutation spectrum

The mutation types in ETV6-related thrombocytopenia with predisposition to malignancies include nonsense, missense, splice site, and frameshift variants. The majority of mutations cluster within the ETS DNA-binding domain and are predicted to be deleterious. The p214L mutation, which resides in the linker region, has been recurrently identified in different families [45, 49].

3.5 Second-hit mutations in ETV6 deficiency

The development of leukemia with variable latency and incomplete penetrance suggests a need for further somatic mutations. Studies did not reveal mutations in the remaining wild-type ETV6 allele in most cases. Such examples are more of an exception. Acquisition of somatic defects in other genes, such as RUNX1, BCOR, and KRAS, is more prominent. The role of additional mutations in malignant transformation remains to be determined [45].

3.6 Molecular structure and role of ETV6

ETV6 is a part of a 26-member family of transcriptional regulators, defined by a highly conserved 85-amino-acid residue that mediates binding of target DNA. Different ETS factors can replace each other in the context of overexpression in vitro but exhibit functional diversity and individual specificity in DNA binding beyond the core motif. ETV6 has the capacity to form polymers with head-to-tail binding of two different protein surfaces within its PNT domain [51].

The primary function of ETV6 is a transcriptional repressor. The PNT domain-mediated multimerization is required for high affinity DNA binding. Truncated ETV6 proteins resulting from frameshift mutations retaining either the PNT domain or the ETS domain were shown to exhibit a dominant-negative activity. This was also demonstrated for the familial germline mutations. This may suggest that the pathogenic activity of ETV6 mutations not only includes loss of function but also interferes with the wild-type allele [40, 52, 53].

ETV6 also plays an important role in embryonic development. Homozygous ETV6 germline disruption results in embryonic lethality in mice studies [54]. ETV6 is required for survival of hematopoietic stem cells in the bone marrow. It also promotes the late phases of megakaryopoiesis. Heterozygous disruption of ETV6 in mice is not associated with obvious phenotypes, implying the dominant-negative effect of germline mutations found in affected families: complete loss of ETV6 is lethal, but development of abnormalities requires more than heterozygous loss [55, 56].

3.7 Clinical management

Treatment of ETV6-related leukemia does not differ from standard protocols. As in FDP-MM, if a disease-causing germline mutation is known in the family, it is necessary to test siblings, as HSCT from a sibling carrier of ETV6 pathogenic variant should be avoided. Family members should be tested, and regular follow-up of mutation carriers including differential blood count is advised. Bone marrow aspiration and/or biopsy with thorough cytogenetic/molecular genetic investigation may be necessary in case of additional cytopenias or other suspicious clinical symptoms [13].

3.8 Conclusion

Discovery of familial ETV6 germline mutations has established its clinical significance as a cause of thrombocytopenia, as well as a major cancer predisposition gene, associated with a substantial number of childhood B-ALL cases as well as myeloid malignancies. However, our understanding of the clinical impact of ETV6 mutations and physiological role of ETV6 remains incomplete. More work is needed to understand the molecular pathology of the mutations and stratify the risk of affected individuals.

4. ANKRD26-related thrombocytopenia

Thrombocytopenia 2 (THC2 MIM 188000) is one of the rarest forms of autosomal-dominant thrombocytopenia. It has so far been reported only in 21 families across the world [57]. The THC2 locus was mapped to chromosome 10p11.1-p12 through linkage analysis in two independent studies [58, 59]. In the original studies, two missense changes in different linked genes were found to be causative of the disease: c.501G > C (p.Glu167Asp) and c.22 C > T (p.his8Tyr). Another study identified pedigrees with six additional ANKRD26 mutations, segregating with thrombocytopenia. All of them were located in a stretch of 19 nucleotides of the 5′ UTR that is highly conserved in evolution. These findings associate ANKRD26 5 ′ UTR mutations with thrombocytopenia [60]. Further reports extended the number of known families to 21 [61]. The abovementioned studies also found that the number of hematologic malignancies was higher than expected.

4.1 Diagnostic criteria, platelet features

THC2-affected individuals have a degree of thrombocytopenia ranging from mild to severe and suffer from a mild bleeding diathesis. Major bleeding events are rare. Platelets are normal-sized and morphology does not reveal any defects. Examination of bone marrow shows dysmegakaryocytopoietic phenomena. No other changes in blood count, e.g., anemia and neutropenia, were reported [60].

4.2 Risk of malignancy

A comprehensive study of 118 subjects affected with THC2 identified 10 patients who developed myeloid malignancies: four acute myeloid leukemias (AML), four myelodysplastic syndromes, and two chronic myeloid leukemias (CML). Cumulative incidence of hematological malignancies in this subset of patients is 8.47%. The incidence of lymphoproliferative disorders and nonhematologic cancers was not higher than expected. Available data are compatible with the hypothesis that ANKRD26-related thrombocytopenia predisposes to myeloid malignancy. However, penetrance for neoplasia is incomplete, and other genetic or environmental factors must contribute to development of these disorders [57].

4.3 Molecular genetics

ANKRD26 is the ancestor of a family of primate-specific genes termed POTE (prostate-ovary-testes- and placenta-expressed genes) whose expression is restricted to several normal to a few normal tissues and a larger number of malignancies, such as breast cancer. ANKRD26 is expressed also in megakaryocytes and to lesser extent erythroid cells [62, 63].

The functional role of ANKRD26 is unknown. Deleterious mutations of aNKRD26 in animal studies do not cause thrombocytopenia. This evidence suggests that THC2 is more likely to be caused by gain-of-function mutations rather than haploinsufficiency. It is suspected that mutations in the 5′ UTR interfere with mechanisms controlling the expression of ANKRD26 and affect megakaryopoiesis and platelet production, possibly by induction of apoptosis [60, 64].

4.4 Clinical management

As in the abovementioned entities, screening for ANKRD26 mutations must be a part of diagnostic process in hereditary thrombocytopenia and familial myeloid leukemia. Follow-up of asymptomatic mutation carriers in regular intervals including peripheral blood count and smear is necessary. The presence of ANKRD26 germline mutations in acute leukemia may also play a part in HSCT-related questions.

4.5 Conclusions

ANKRD26 is a rare form of inherited thrombocytopenia with low risk of bleeding and predisposition to myeloid malignancies. Recognition of this disorder is important in differential diagnosis of hereditary thrombocytopenia and proper management of affected subjects.

5. Further candidate genes

There are several genes associated with inherited bone marrow failure syndromes (IBMFS) and thrombocytopenia, notably MPL, THPO, HOXA11, MECOM, and RBM8A, as well as mutations in genes for X-linked thrombocytopenia and immune deficiency (GATA1, WAS) [65]. These clinical entities present with thrombopenia or pancytopenia and, in some cases, dysmorphic features. The IBMFS are complex disorders unified by development of bone marrow failure and increased risk of leukemic transformation. In some IBMFS, the steps toward leukemic transformation are better understood. In others, there is still much to learn. The estimated risk of malignancy in the abovementioned entities requires additional research.

MYH9 mutations result in congenital macrothrombocytopenia and predispose to kidney failure, hearing loss, and cataracts. There are a few published cases of germline mutations of MYH9 with myeloid malignancy [66]. Somatic expression of MYH9 has impact on overall survival in patients with AML [67]. However, additional studies on larger patient populations are needed to confirm this suspicion.

6. Conclusion

In this chapter, we have summarized current knowledge of familial syndromes with thrombocytopenia and predisposition to hematologic malignancies. These rare disorders must be a part of differential diagnosis of (1) unexplained or familial thrombocytopenia, (2) myeloid malignancies with familial occurrence, and (3) bone marrow failure syndromes. Only a correct diagnosis with up-to-date hematological and molecular diagnostics can lead to proper follow-up of affected individuals and families. Personalized risk assessment must be made; and in the case of a familial germline mutation, genetic reproductive consultation should be offered.

Acknowledgements

This text was created with the help of my supervisor, Prof. Michael Doubek, MD, and colleagues from Department of Internal Medicine, Hematology and Oncology, Central European Institute of Technology.

This text was produced with the help of "Pomoc lidem s leukémií" foundation. This work was supported by Czech Ministry of Health (grant AZV 16-29447A) and Masaryk University (grant MUNI/A/1105/2018).

Conflict of interest

The authors declare no conflict of interest.

Author details

Jakub Trizuljak[1,2]* and Michael Doubek[1,2]

1 Central European Institute of Technology (CEITEC), Masaryk University, Brno, Czech Republic

2 Department of Internal Medicine—Hematology and Oncology, University Hospital and Masaryk University, Brno, Czech Republic

*Address all correspondence to: trizuljak.jakub@fnbrno.cz

References

[1] Fanconi G. Familiäre infantile perniziosaartige Anämie (perniziöses Blutbild und Konstitution). Jahrbuch Kinderheilk. 1927;**117**:257-280

[2] Wlodarski MW, Niemeyer CM. Introduction: Genetic syndromes predisposing to myeloid neoplasia. Seminars in Hematology. 2017;**54**(2):57-59. DOI: 10.1053/j.seminhematol.2017.05.001

[3] Pecci A. Diagnosis and treatment of inherited thrombocytopenias. Clinical Genetics. 2016;**89**(2):141-153

[4] Arber DA, Orazi A, Hasserijan R, et al. The 2016 revision to the World Health Organization classification of myeloid neoplasms and acute leukemia. Blood. 2016;**127**(20):2391-2405. DOI: 10.1182/blood-2016-03-643544

[5] Schlegelberger B, Heller PG. *RUNX1* deficiency (familial platelet disorder with predisposition to myeloid leukemia, FPDMM). Seminars in Hematology. 2017;**54**(2):75-80. DOI: 10.1053/j.seminhematol.2017.04.006

[6] Hayashi Y, Harada Y, Huang G, Harada H. Myeloid neoplasms with germ line *RUNX1* mutation. International Journal of Hematology. 2017;**106**(2):183-188. DOI: 10.1007/s12185-017-2258-5

[7] Osato M, Asou N, Abdalla E, Hoshino K, Yamasaki H, Okubo T, et al. Biallelic and heterozygous point mutations in the runt domain of the AML1/PEBP2alphaB gene associated with myeloblastic leukemias. Blood. 1999;**93**(6):1817-1824

[8] Song WJ, Sullivan MG, Legare RD, Hutchings S, Tan X, Kufrin D, et al. Haploinsufficiency of CBFA2 causes familial thrombocytopenia with propensity to develop acute myelogenous leukaemia. Nature Genetics. 1999;**23**(2):166-175. DOI: 10.1038/13793

[9] Churpek JE, Godley LA. How I diagnose and manage individuals at risk for inherited myeloid malignancies. Blood. 2016;**128**(14):1800-1813. DOI: 10.1182/blood-2016-05-670240

[10] Latger-Cannard V, Philippe C, Bouquet A, et al. Haematological spectrum and genotype-phenotype correlations in nine unrelated families with RUNX1 mutations from the French network on inherited platelet disorders. Orphanet Journal of Rare Diseases. 2016;**11**:49. DOI: 10.1186/s13023-016-0432-0

[11] Braddock SR, South ST, Schiffman JD, Longhurst M, Rowe LR, Carey JC. Braddock-Carey syndrome: A 21q22 contiguous gene syndrome encompassing RUNX1. American Journal of Medical Genetics. Part A. 2016;**170**(10):2580-2586. DOI: 10.1002/ajmg.a.37870

[12] Ripperger T, Tauscher M, Thomay K, et al. No evidence for ITSN1 loss in a patient with mental retardation and complex chromosomalr earrangements of 21q21-21q22. Leukemia Research 2013;**37**(6):721-723. DOI: 10.1016/j.leukres.2013.02.013

[13] Churpek JE, Lorenz R, Nedumgottil S, et al. Proposal for the clinical detection and management of patients and their family members with familial myelodysplastic syndrome/acute leukemia predisposition syndromes. Leukemia & Lymphoma. 2013;**54**(1):28-35. DOI: 10.3109/10428194.2012.701738

[14] Kozubík KS, Radová L, Pešová M, Réblová K, Trizuljak J, Plevová K, et al. C-terminal RUNX1 mutation in familial platelet disorder with predisposition to myeloid malignancies. International Journal

of Hematology. 2018;**108**(6):652-657. DOI: 10.1007/s12185-018-2514-3. Epub 2018 Aug 6

[15] Babushok DV, Bessler M. Genetic predisposition syndromes: When should they be considered in the work-up of MDS? Best Practice & Research. Clinical Haematology. 2015;**28**(1):55-68. DOI: 10.1016/j.beha.2014.11.004

[16] Owen C, Barnett M, Fitzgibbon J. Familial myelodysplasia and acute myeloid leukaemia—A review. British Journal of Haematology. 2008;**140**:123-132. DOI: 10.1111/j.1365-2141.2007.06909.x

[17] Ripperger T, Tawana K, Kratz C, Schlegelberger B, Fitzgibbon J, Steinemann D. Clinical utility gene card for: Familial platelet disorder with associated myeloid malignancies. European Journal of Human Genetics. 2016;**24**:1232. DOI: 10.1038/ejhg.2015.278

[18] Preudhomme C, Renneville A, Bourdon V, et al. High frequency of RUNX1 biallelic alteration in acute myeloid leukemia secondary to familial platelet disorder. Blood. 2009;**113**(22):5583-5587. DOI: 10.1182/blood-2008-07-168260

[19] Noris P, Biino G, Pecci A, et al. Platelet diameters in inherited thrombocytopenias: Analysis of 376 patients with all known disorders. Blood. 2014;**124**(6):e4-e10. DOI: 10.1182/blood-2014-03-564328

[20] Bluteau D, Glembotsky AC, Raimbault A, et al. Dysmegakaryopoiesis of FPD/AML pedigrees with constitutional RUNX1 mutations is linked to myosin II deregulated expression. Blood. 2012;**120**(13):2708-2718. DOI: 10.1182/blood-2012-04-422337

[21] Glembotsky AC, Bluteau D, Espasandin YR, et al. Mechanisms underlying platelet function defect in a pedigree with familial platelet disorder with a predisposition to acute myelogenous leukemia: Potential role for candidate RUNX1 targets. Journal of Thrombosis and Haemostasis. 2014;**12**(5):761-772. DOI: 10.1111/jth.12550

[22] Heller PG, Glembotsky AC, Gandhi MJ, et al. Low Mpl receptor expression in a pedigree with familial platelet disorder with predisposition to acute myelogenous leukemia and a novel AML1 mutation. Blood. 2005;**105**(12):4664-4670. DOI: 10.1182/blood-2005-01-0050

[23] Kaur G, Jalagadugula G, Mao G, Rao AK. RUNX1/core binding factor A2 Regulates platelet 12-lipoxygenasegene (ALOX12): Studies in human RUNX1 haplodeficiency. Blood. 2010;**115**:3128-3135. DOI: 10.1182/blood-2009-04-214601

[24] Antony-Debre I, Bluteau D, Itzykson R, et al. MYH10 protein expression in platelets as a biomarker of RUNX1 and FLI1 alterations. Blood. 2012;**120**(13):2719-2722. DOI: 10.1182/blood-2012-04-422352

[25] Ng KP, Hu Z, Ebrahem Q, Negrotto S, Lausen J, Saunthararajah Y. Runx1 deficiency permits granulocyte lineage commitment but impairs subsequent maturation. Oncogene. 2013;**2**:e78. DOI: 10.1038/oncsis.2013.41

[26] Satoh Y, Matsumura I, Tanaka H, et al. C-terminal mutation of RUNX1 attenuates the DNA-damage repair response in hematopoietic stem cells. Leukemia. 2012;**26**(2):303-311. DOI: 10.1038/leu.2011.202

[27] Kirito K, Mitsumori T, Nagashima T, et al. A novel inherited single-nucleotide mutation in50-UTR in the transcription factor RUNX1 in familial platelet disorder with propensity to develop myeloid malignancies. Blood 2006;**108**:1917. http://www.bloodjournal.org/content/108/11/1917

[28] Antony-Debre I, Manchev VT, Balayn N, et al. Level of RUNX1 activity is critical for leukemic predisposition but not for thrombocytopenia. Blood. 2015;**125**(6):930-940. DOI: 10.1182/blood-2014-06-585513

[29] Ripperger T, Tauscher M, Ehlert L, et al. Childhood onset of leukaemia in familial platelet disorder with propensity for myeloid malignancies due to an intragenic RUNX1 deletion. Haematologica. 2012;**97**:s3-S14

[30] Churpek JE, Pyrtel K, Kanchi KL, et al. Genomic analysis of germline and somatic variants in familial myelodysplasia/acute myeloid leukemia. Blood. 2015;**126**:2484-2490. DOI: 10.1182/blood-2015-04-641100

[31] Sakurai M, Kasahara H, Yoshida K, et al. Genetic basis of myeloid transformation in familial platelet disorder/acute myeloid leukemia patients with haploinsufficient RUNX1 allele. Blood Cancer Journal. 2016;**6**:e392. DOI: 10.1002/gcc.21918

[32] Haferlach C, Bacher U, Schnittger S, et al. ETV6 rearrangements are recurrent in myeloid malignancies and are frequently associated with other genetic events. Genes, Chromosomes & Cancer. 2012;**51**:328-337. DOI: 10.1002/gcc.21918

[33] Yoshimi A, ToyaT KM, et al. Recurrent CDC25C mutations drive malignant transformation in FPD/AML. Nature Communications. 2014;**5**:4770. DOI: 10.1038/ncomms5770

[34] Haslam K, Langabeer SE, Hayat A, Conneally E, Vandenberghe E. Targeted next-generation sequencing of familial platelet disorder with predisposition to acute myeloid leukaemia. British Journal of Haematology. 2016;**175**:161-163. DOI: 10.1111/bjh.13838

[35] Golub TR, Barker GF, Lovett M, Gilliland DG. Fusion of PDGF receptor beta to a novel ets-like gene, tel, in chronic myelomonocytic leukemia with t(5;12) chromosomal translocation. Cell. 1994;77(2):307-316

[36] de Braekeleer E, Auffret R, Garcia JR, Padilla JM, Fletes CC, Morel F, et al. Identification of NIPBL, a new ETV6 partner gene in t(5;12) (p13;p13)-associated acute megakaryoblastic leukemia. Leukemia & Lymphoma. 2013;**54**(2):423-424. DOI: 10.3109/10428194.2012.706288

[37] Hollenhorst PC, McIntosh LP, Graves BJ. Genomic and biochemical insights into the specificity of ETS transcription factors. Annual Review of Biochemistry. 2011;**80**:437-471. DOI: 10.1146/annurev.biochem.79.081507.103945

[38] De Braekeleer E, Douet-Guilbert N, Morel F, Le Bris MJ, Basinko A, De Braekeleer M. ETV6 fusion genes in hematological malignancies: A review. Leukemia Research. 2012;**36**(8):945-961. DOI: 10.1016/j.leukres.2012.04.010

[39] Papaemmanuil E. RapadoI, Li Y, et al. RAG-mediated recombination is the predominant driver of oncogenic rearrangement in ETV6-RUNX1 acute lymphoblastic leukemia. Nature Genetics. 2014;**46**(2):116-125. DOI: 10.1038/ng.2874

[40] van Doorn SB, Spensberger D, de Knegt Y, Tang M, Spensberger D, et al. Somatic heterozygous mutations in ETV6 (TEL) and frequent absence of ETV6 protein in acute myeloid leukemia. Oncogene. 2005;**24**(25): 4129-4137. DOI: 10.1038/sj.onc.1208588

[41] Van Vlierberghe P, Ambesi-Impiombato A, Perez-Garcia A, et al. ETV6 mutations in early immature human T cell leukemias. The Journal of Experimental Medicine. 2011;**208**(13):2571-2579. DOI: 10.1084/jem.20112239

[42] Zhang J, Ding L, Holmfeldt L, et al. The genetic basis of early T-cell precursor acute lymphoblastic leukaemia. Nature. 2012;**481**(7380): 157-163. DOI: 10.1038/nature10725

[43] Zhang J, Mullighan CG, Harvey RC, et al. Key pathways are frequently mutated in high-risk childhood acute lymphoblastic leukemia: A report from the children's oncology group. Blood. 2011;**118**(11):3080-3087. DOI: 10.1182/blood-2011-03-341412

[44] Lohr JG, Stojanov P, Lawrence MS, et al. Discovery and prioritization of somatic mutations in diffuse large B-cell lymphoma (DLBCL) by whole-exome sequencing. Proceedings of the National Academy of Sciences of the United States of America. 2012;**109**(10): 3879-3884. DOI: 10.1073/pnas.1121343109

[45] Zhang MY, Churpek JE, Keel SB, et al. Germline ETV6 mutations in familial thrombocytopenia and hematologic malignancy. Nature Genetics. 2015;**47**(2). DOI: 10.1038/ng.3177

[46] Noetzli L, Lo RW, Lee-Sherick AB, et al. Germline mutations inETV6 are associated with thrombocytopenia, red cell macrocytosis and predisposition to lymphoblastic leukemia. Nature Genetics. 2015;**47**(5):535-538. DOI: 10.1038/ng.3253

[47] Melazzini F, Palombo F, Balduini A, Doubek M, et al. Clinical and pathogenic features of ETV6-related thrombocytopenia with predisposition to acute lymphoblastic leukemia. Haematologica. 2016;**101**(11):1333-1342. 0-5. DOI: 10.3324/haematol.2016.147496

[48] Poggi M, Canault M, Favier M, et al. Germline variants in ETV6 underlie reduced platelet formation, platelet dysfunction and increased levels of circulating CD34+ progenitors. Haematologica. 2017;**102**(2):282-294. DOI: 10.3324/haematol.2016.147694

[49] Moriyama T, Metzger ML, Wu G, et al. Germline genetic variation in ETV6 and risk of childhood acute lymphoblastic leukaemia: A systematic genetic study. The Lancet Oncology. 2015;**16**(16):1659-1666. DOI: 10.1016/S1470-2045(15)00369-1

[50] Topka S, Vijai J, Walsh MF, et al. Germline ETV6 mutations confer susceptibility to acute lymphoblastic leukemia and thrombocytopenia. PLoS Genetics. 2015;**11**(6):e1005262. DOI: 10.1371/journal.pgen.1005262

[51] Wasylyk C, Maira SM, Sobieszczuk P, Wasylyk B. Reversion of Ras transformed cells by ETS transdominant mutants. Oncogene. 1994;**9**(12):3665-3673

[52] Fenrick R, Wang L, Nip J, et al. TEL, a putative tumor suppressor, modulates cell growth and cell morphology of ras-transformed cells while repressing the transcription of stromelysin-1. Molecular and Cellular Biology. 2000;**20**(16):5828-5839

[53] Park H, Seo Y, Kim JI, Kim WJ, Choe SY. Identification of the nuclear localization motif in the ETV6 (TEL) protein. Cancer Genetics and Cytogenetics. 2006;**167**(2):117-121. DOI: 10.1016/j.cancergencyto.2006.01.006

[54] Wang LC, Kuo F, Fujiwara Y, Gilliland DG, Golub TR, Orkin SH. Yolk sac angiogenic defect and intra-embryonic apoptosis in mice lacking the Ets-related factor TEL. The EMBO Journal. 1997;**16**(14):4374-4383. DOI: 10.1093/emboj/16.14.4374

[55] Hock H, Meade E, Medeiros S, et al. Tel/Etv6 is an essential and selective regulator of adult hematopoietic stem cell survival. Genes & Development. 2004;**18**(19):2336-2341. DOI: 10.1101/gad.1239604

[56] Wang LC, Swat W, Fujiwara Y, et al. The TEL/ETV6 gene is required

specifically for hematopoiesis in the bone marrow. Genes & Development. 1998;**12**(15):2392-2402. DOI: 10.1101/gad.12.15.2392

[57] Noris P, Favier R, Alessi MC, Geddis AE, Kunishima S, Heller PG, et al. *ANKRD26*-related thrombocytopenia and myeloid malignancies. Blood. 2013;**122**(11):1987-1989. DOI: 10.1182/blood-2013-04-499319

[58] Savoia A, Del Vecchio M, Totaro A, Perrotta S, Amendola G, Moretti A, et al. An autosomal dominant thrombocytopenia gene maps to chromosomal region 10p. American Journal of Human Genetics. 1999;**65**:1401-1405. DOI: 10.1086/302637

[59] Drachman JG, Jarvik GP, Mehaffey MG. Autosomal dominant thrombocytopenia: Incomplete megakaryocyte differentiation and linkage to human chromosome 10. Blood. 2000;**96**:118-125

[60] Pippucci T, Savoia A, Perrotta S, et al. Mutations in the 5' UTR of ANKRD26, the ankirin repeat domain 26 gene, cause an autosomal-dominant form of inherited thrombocytopenia, THC2. American Journal of Human Genetics. 2011;**88**(1):115-120. DOI: 10.1016/j.ajhg.2010.12.006

[61] Noris P, Perrotta S, Seri M, et al. Mutations in ANKRD26 are responsible for a frequent form of inherited thrombocytopenia: Analysis of 78 patients from 21 families. Blood. 2011;**117**(24):6673-6680. DOI: 10.1182/blood-2011-02-336537

[62] Hahn Y, Bera TK, Pastan IH, Lee B. Duplication and extensive remodeling shaped POTE family genes encoding proteins containing ankyrin repeat and coiled coil domains. Gene. 2006;**366**:238-245. DOI: 10.1016/j.gene.2005.07.045

[63] Macaulay IC, Tijssen MR, Thijssen-Timmer DC, Gusnanto A, Steward M, Burns P, et al. Comparative gene expression profiling of in vitro differentiated megakaryocytes and erythroblasts identifies novel activatory and inhibitory platelet membrane proteins. Blood. 2007;**109**:3260-3269. DOI: 10.1182/blood-2006-07-036269

[64] Bera TK, Liu XF, Yamada M, Gavrilova O, Mezey E, Tessarollo L, et al. A model for obesity and gigantism due to disruption of the Ankrd26 gene. Proceedings of the National Academy of Sciences. 2008;**105**:270-275. DOI: 10.1073/pnas.0710978105

[65] Bluteau O et al. A landscape of germ line mutations in a cohort of inherited bone marrow failure patients. Blood; Feb 15 2018;**131**(7):717-732. DOI: 10.1182/blood-2017-09-806489

[66] Rheingold SR. Acute myeloid leukemia in a child with hereditary thrombocytopenia. Pediatric Blood & Cancer. 2007;**48**(1):105-107. DOI: 10.1002/pbc.20677

[67] Yu M, Wang J, Zhu Z, et al. Prognostic impact of MYH9 expression on patients with acute myeloid leukemia. Oncotarget. 2016;**8**(1):156-163. DOI: 10.18632/oncotarget.10613

Section 4

Energy Failure and Leukemia

Chapter 4

Perturbations in Generation and Flow of Energy in the Eukaryotic Cell Explain the Chromosomal Instability Syndrome

Arturo Solis Herrera

Abstract

Chromosomal instability is poorly defined and used inconsistently and imprecisely. It is the increased propensity to chromosome aberrations due to chromosome replication, repair, or segregation. Therefore, acquired genetic changes are central to leukemia development. Fast-growing cells require substantive amount of energy; however, tumor cells take up more glucose, processing it through aerobic glycolysis producing large lactate amounts with lower use of oxidative phosphorylation to generate ATP. The Warburg effect is characterized by reduced use of tricarboxylic acid cycle, so pyruvate made in glycolysis is converted into lactate and expelled, but this metabolic pathway is energetically inefficient. When genes are malfunctioning, both oncogenes and tumor suppressor genes influence negatively the switch between aerobic glycolysis and extensive use of TCA cycle to generate ATP, as the normal gene replication and expression require adequate energy levels. Chromosomal instability is increasingly entangled and unnecessarily complex. So far, researchers focused solely on studying the mass and have forgotten the energy. The intrinsic property of melanin to transform light into chemical energy, through water dissociation, as chlorophyll in plants, opens a new landscape in chromosome biology, highlighting the role of the environment toxics in leukemia pathogenesis, inhalation being the dominant pathway of exposure.

Keywords: energy, chromosome instability, hydrogen, oxygen, melanin, water dissociation, benzene

1. Introduction

Chromosomic instability is characterized by aneuploidy, allelic losses, and the consecutive accumulation of chromosomal abnormalities [1].

Aneuploidy is widely acknowledged as a leading cause of miscarriage and birth defects in humans and is generally known to be deleterious to the survival of individual cells. However, aneuploidy is also ubiquitous in cancer and is thought to arise as an adaptive response in certain contexts given the technical difficulties to study it and the poor understanding of the involved processes. This dichotomy of aneuploidy has attracted the interest of researchers for over a century, but many studies have reached conflicting conclusions [2] which reflect how difficult it is to understand billions of years of evolution. The emergence of new technology apparently has allowed scientists to revisit the aneuploidy problem and has fueled several recent studies aimed at understanding the effects of aneuploidy on cell physiology with frustrating results. Therefore, the reviewing of those studies, considering previous observations and knowledge, specifically focusing on the effects of aneuploidy on cellular homeostasis, chromosome stability, and adaptation, gives notably fewer useful conclusions than the expected.

Under normal conditions, genomic integrity is given by chromosomes that are assembled by the DNA sequence and proteins, such as histones that play essential structural and functional roles in the transition between active and inactive chromatin states [3]. Histones have a high degree of conservation regarding maintaining the overall structure of the nucleosomal octameric core.

The DNA is hierarchically packed in the nucleus with the aid of proteins forming a complex called chromatin. Histone variants and posttranslational modifications and interactions with chromatin remodeling complexes influence DNA replication, transcription, repair, and recombination.

The study of the chromatin has been focused in the structural aspect only. And even this type of analysis faces, so far, formidable technical challenges. But it's not simple or even possible to find articles about the flow of energy through the nucleus, nor works on the absence of mitochondria and ATP in the cell nucleus.

Despite the progress in structural studies, we cannot yet answer the question of who controls who. Does chromatin control histones or vice versa or both or other genetic or epigenetic factors?

Eukaryotic chromatin is a highly dynamic macromolecular assembly, which means that it requires energy expenditure continuously, not only to carry out its functions but also to preserve the shape of each component, beginning with the covalent bonds and other types in every molecule, and so on until it reaches to the macromolecule. Most eukaryotic organisms have multiple copies of histone gene; thereby, they are highly conserved in evolution.

The highly complex histone interactions with the nucleosomal core particle are processes that happen in amazing accurate way. All histone domains share a similar structural motif; they form interfaces with each other in several unique ways. This interface specificity is consistent across many variant histone sequences, demonstrating the flexible and adaptable architecture of histone complexes. These are extraordinarily complex biochemical processes that repeat in the same way since the beginning of time.

So far, it is not clear if chromatin inactivation is due to an enzymatic activity and/or a steric block that impedes access by transcription factors or the chromatin remodeling machinery [4]. However, there is an unexpected actor that has not been studied at least in detail: the generation and distribution or flow of energy (from melanin) across the cell nucleus.

It is relatively easy to reverse core histone tails, i.e., by acetylation, methylation, ubiquitination, and phosphorylation, among others [5]. So it is interesting the evolution could happen relatively fast. Evolution is not a process of trial and error, because in that way it would have required time lapse greater than the age of the universe.

Thereby it is possible that the generation and distribution of energy coming from melanin not only releases energy but also is giving information.

1.1 Chromosomal instability

CIN is a form of genomic instability in which chromosomes are uneven, such that either whole chromosomes or fractions of chromosomes are duplicated or deleted. The inadequate distribution of DNA to daughter cells upon mitosis results in a failure to maintain euploidy (the correct number of chromosomes) leading to aneuploidy (incorrect number of chromosomes). The daughter cells do not have the same number of chromosomes as the cell they originated from.

In solid and hematological cancers, chromosomal instability is a common occurrence [6], involving gain or loss of whole chromosomes or fraction of chromosomes [7]. Chromosomal instability is thought to be an early event during tumorigenesis or furthermore is involved in tumor initiation.

Cancers result from the accumulation of inherited and somatic mutations in oncogenes and tumor suppressor genes [8]. Supposedly, these genes encode proteins that function in growth regulatory and differentiation pathways. Mutations in those genes increase the net reproductive rate of cells. Mutations in genes increase the rate at which whole chromosomes or large parts of chromosomes are lost or gained during cell division.

Chromosomal instability causes an imbalance in chromosome number (aneuploidy) and an enhanced rate of loss of heterozygosity, which seems as an important mechanism of inactivating tumor suppressor genes. Thereby, cancer results if normal regulatory mechanisms of cell birth and death are disrupted [9].

Maintenance of chromosomal stability requires a statistically nonsignificant gene mutation. Many cancers, if not all, are characterized by a high degree of aneuploidy, result of chromosomal instability mainly. However, linear analysis of chromosomal instability with mathematical models suggests that it does not arise simply because it allows a faster accumulation of carcinogenic mutations. Instead chromosomal instability must arise because other reasons, such as environmental factors, epigenetic events, or as direct consequence of a tumor suppressor gene inactivation. The increased variability alone is not enough explanation for the presence of chromosomal instability in most cancers [10].

The characteristics of cancer cells as aneuploidy, and multiple chromosomal anomalies including gain or loss of whole chromosomes or transposed chromosomal fragments [11], suggest that many cell processes are failing at the same time. The above is compatible with a generalized failure, which is characteristic of energy problems.

The prior intracellular conditions necessary to induce substantive mutations in the genes as well as aneuploidy, which are considered necessary conditions for neoplastic transformation; they are like widespread chaos inside the cell. And in a biological system as evolved as the eukaryote, cell is difficult to explain, unless we take energy into account.

Maybe, so far, the investigation did not consider the energy flow required by the cell nucleus because it does not have mitochondria or ATP. And perhaps that's why you might think it does not require energy; but the cell nucleus is the largest intracellular organelle, so its energy needs are expected to be substantive; and on the other hand, let us remember that the cell uses energy in many ways, not only to impel each and every one of the amazingly accurate biochemical reactions that make up what we call life, which happen in the same way, with the same sequence, with the same temporality, with the same molecules, with the same location, and in similar proportions since the beginning of the time.

We can think that the eukaryotic cell knows his work perfectly, because he has done it millions of years, millions of times. But the astonishing perfection and characteristic coordination of living entities requires a source of energy that possesses similar characteristics, which are so different from the ATP energy currency prevalent theory.

The cell, therefore, requires energy for many things, not only to carry out the extraordinarily complex biological functions that we are far from understanding but even to preserve the form and stability.

1.2 Hematopoietic stem cell

The biochemical processes involved with the hematopoiesis are extraordinarily complex and surprisingly accurate, since they have been repeated in the same way continually since the beginning of time. They can be disturbed by physicochemical alterations in some of their foremost components, for example, the water viscosity is one of the characteristics that is altered with greatest ease.

The bone marrow produces an average of 2.5 million erythrocytes per second, which requires prodigious amounts of precursors of organic molecules and energy. And the production of such a quantity of blood-forming elements requires great and fast coordination between the different and highly biochemical processes involved, since they must happen with an astonishing exactitude, but their main requirement is, without a doubt, energy.

Hematopoiesis in the bone marrow turns ineffective when the biochemical steps that make up and that happen at a staggering speed suffer some alteration due to the presence of contaminants in water, in the air, or in food such as pesticides, herbicides, fertilizers, metals, plastics, solvents, industrial waste, drugs, anesthetic agents, alcohol, drug addiction, extreme climates (cold, heat) etc.

This perturbed hematopoiesis in the bone marrow can lead to cytopenias in the blood and predisposition to acute myeloid leukemia (AML) [12]. There is a delicate interplay between the hematopoietic stem and progenitor cells, stromal cells, and cytokines or chemokines secreted within the microenvironment that is needed to maintain hematopoiesis. Thereby, this microenvironment is at the same time highly complex and highly dynamic, requiring enough available chemical energy at any moment.

The bone marrow is separated into vascular and nonvascular sections. The vascular section contains blood vessels that supply the bone with nutrients and transport CO_2, blood stem cells, and mature cells away from the bone and into circulation. The nonvascular sections of the bone marrow are where the hematopoiesis or blood cell formation occurs.

It is contradictory that in nonvascular section of bone marrow, hematopoiesis takes place. Supposedly, the current deep-rooted dogma says that our body can get the energy and mass precursors through a single molecule, this is glucose. However, glucose requires to be transported through blood stream, and surprisingly, the bone marrow section with the highest metabolic rate has no blood vessels at all.

Something similar happens in human retina, where the rod and cone layer, with a metabolic rate almost ten times greater than cerebral cortex, under normal conditions, it has no blood vessels at all.

Bone marrow stromal cells are progenitors of skeletal tissue components such as the bone, cartilage, the hematopoiesis-supporting stroma, and adipocytes and possibly can also form neural and myogenic cells [13].

In average, there are 2.5 trillion of red blood cells in your body at any moment. To maintain this number, under normal conditions, about two and a half million new ones need to be produced every second by your bone marrow. Considering all the tissues and cells in our body, 25 million new cells are being produced each second. We give birth to over 200 billion red cells every day.

Hypoxia or low oxygen availability is a prominent molecular feature of the bone marrow that contributes to both normal and malignant hematopoiesis. Relative to most tissues, the bone marrow microenvironment resides in a particularly hypoxic microenvironment. Oxygen tensions within the bone marrow cavity range from 0.6% to 4.2%, whereas oxygen tensions in most other adult tissues range from 2 to 9% O_2 [14]. But because each cell can dissociate the molecule from water, thanks to melanin, then oxygen levels are an indirect indicator of molecular hydrogen levels in tissues.

The purely structural analysis of bone marrow, as it has been to date, confronts, at least two important challenges: (1) substantive technical limitations due to the complex anatomy and biochemistry of the area to study and (2) researchers are trying to decipher 4 billion years of evolution without considering the generation and flow of energy.

1.3 Glucose

Glucose is (supposedly) an important fuel that is used by nearly all organisms through a common set of metabolic pathways. The knowledge of glucose metabolism that is prevalent until today, dates to 1860, with the identification of glycolysis with Louis Pasteur and thereafter in 1937, with the work of Gustav Embden and Otto Fritz Meyerhof [15]. Also, in 1937, the foundations of citric acid cycle were provided by Albert Szent-Gyorgyi, Hans A. Krebs, and William A. Johnson [16]. Two decades later, Peter D. Mitchell hypothesized a chemiosmotic mechanism that supposedly led to the elucidation of the electron transport chain and oxidative phosphorylation [17]. Thereby, at least apparently, the pathway for aerobic glucose metabolism and ATP generation was completed.

However, glucose is the universal precursor of any organic matter in the human body, but it cannot provide the energy that its own metabolism requires. Our circumstantial finding in human retina, during an observational study about the three main worldwide causes of blindness, about the unsuspected intrinsic property of melanin to dissociate the water molecule, like chlorophyll in plants [18], constitutes a disruptive discovery because it destroys existing dogmas deeply rooted and allows to open new ways to knowledge (**Figure 1**).

Glucose and ATP have biological functions related mainly to biomass metabolism and not so much with energy. The unexpected intrinsic property of melanin to transform photon energy into chemical energy through the dissociation of water molecule, a role performed supposedly only by chlorophyll in plants, seriously questions the sacrosanct role of glucose and thereby mitochondria and ATP as the primary source of energy for the cells (**Figure 2**). Furthermore, increased glycosylation has been linked to increased apoptosis [19].

If we accepted by a moment that our body is able to take energy from the light thanks to the melanin, then the absence of blood vessels in anatomical structures with very high metabolic rate such as photoreceptors of the retina and the avascular region of the bone marrow is now explainable, and it is congruent with the fact that the blood vessels are not able to transport energy (**Figures 3** and **4**).

The absence of capillaries in anatomical regions with a high metabolic cup is explained, at least, for two reasons:

A. Blood cannot carry on energy. The bloodstream only transports metabolites and their intermediaries. Considering the discovery of the unsuspected bioenergetic role of melanin, the main gas that the blood transports is the CO_2. Recall that unknowns about blood are important and numerous, for example, albumin formula is not yet known, and by other side, the similitudes of hemoglobin and chlorophyll molecules are substantive, thereby cannot be discarded that hemoglobin can also dissociate the water molecule, irreversible, like chlorophyll.

B. If all the capillaries in the human body were lined up in a single file, the line would stretch over 100,000 miles. It's been estimated that there are 40 billion capillaries in the average human body.

The circulatory system has a complex design and is very extensive, and not all capillaries are permeable at the same time, supposedly something less than half is

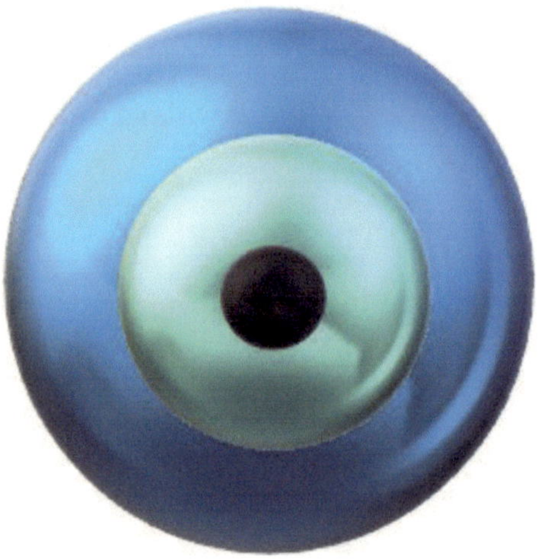

Figure 1.
Schematic representation of the way in which melanin (center) dissipates the energy it absorbs, dissociating the water molecule, that is, hydrogen and molecular oxygen (H_2 and O_2), which are released in the form of growing spheres of energy that follow the laws of simple diffusion. The difference in color of the spheres is to remark that a sphere contains higher concentration of H_2 and O_2, result of the dissociation of the water; the next sphere would contain higher quantity of electrons of high energy, as melanin generates four electrons of high energy for every two molecules of water that is reassociated.

Plants:

$$2H_2O \rightarrow 2H_2 + O_2$$

Humans:

$$2H_2O \rightarrow 2H_2 + O_2 \rightarrow 2H_2O + 4e^-$$

Figure 2.
General outline of the very first step in photosynthesis in plants and humans. In plants the chlorophyll dissociates irreversibly the water molecule by expelling the oxygen to the atmosphere. In humans, melanin dissociates the water molecule in reversible form, and for every two water molecules that are reformed, four high-energy electrons are generated.

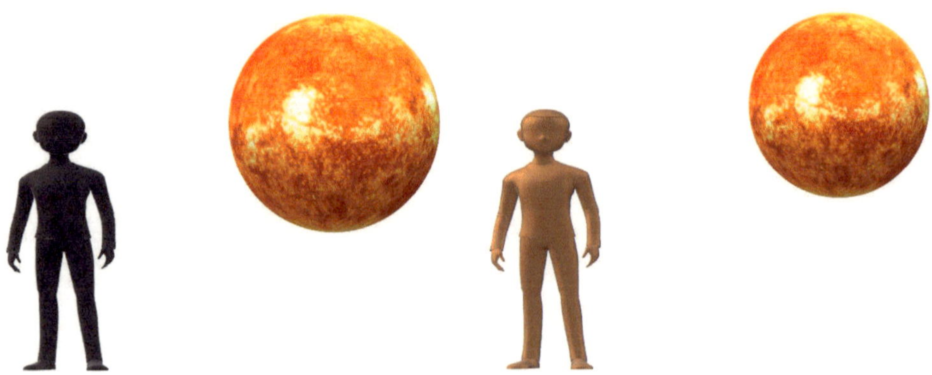

Figure 3.
When the amount of sunlight is abundant, as in the tropics, the amount of melanin in the skin is higher to regulate the quantity of light that must penetrate the inside of the organism, because even the bone marrow requires luminous energy continuously. It is not surprising that leukemia in white people is more frequent than in dark-skinned people.

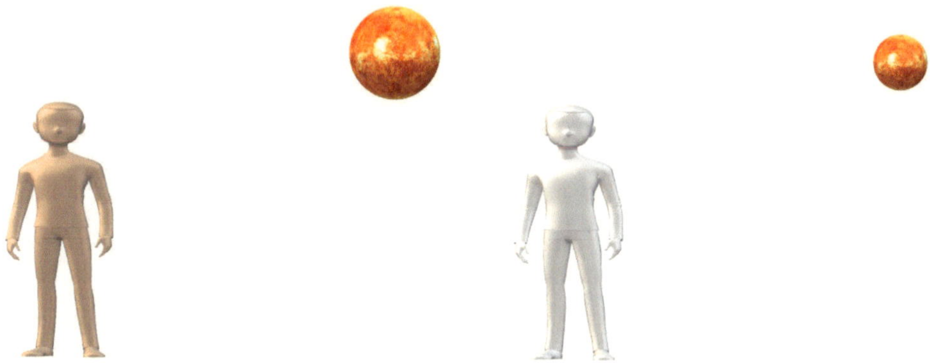

Figure 4.
When the amount of sunlight is lower, as in cold countries, the amount of melanin in the skin decreases to allow for a greater passage of light, and in that way, the final quantity of light that the body inside needs will remain the right one. The amount of melanin in the skin is determined by the amount of light in the environment where people inhabit.

closed at a given time, otherwise, the volume of circulating blood would not reach to fill them all at the same time.

The intricate circulatory system and its highly complex blood content have functions related to the biology of the structure or mass mainly, but anyway energy expenditure is constantly required, thereby, our body or the cell itself, can capture it from visible and invisible light, and it is transduced into chemical energy by melanin, throughout the dissociation of the water molecule, like chlorophyll in plants and hemoglobin in blood.

Melanin absorbs the full electromagnetic spectrum, visible and invisible light, from radio waves to gamma rays; thereby, the process of transduction is quite similar during night and day, the products being molecular hydrogen (H_2) from water dissociation and high-energy electrons (*e*-) from reformatted water.

The cells are energetically independent, because melanin is found in every one of them, mainly placed in the perinuclear space; therefore, each cell can generate its own energy by dissociating the water molecule (**Figure** 5).

The fact is surprising that in the different schemes of the cell, melanin passes unnoticed, very seldom or never depicted in the drawings of the eukaryotic cell. It is necessary to add the melanosomes in the perinuclear space, its main location (**Figure 6**).

On the other hand, the rarely noticed absence of mitochondria and ATP in the cell nucleus, the largest organelle of the eukaryotic cell, now has a coherence with the presence of melanosomes in the perinuclear space, which surround the nucleus, while they provide it with the energy necessary for its functions (**Figure** 7).

Hence the importance of water in living beings, because it is the perfect substrate for melanin that must always be available and accessible so that the cell can obtain the energy it requires incessantly throught water dissociation.

The water content of the cells is very high, 77% by weight and 94.54% by number of molecules, and the constant need for water (and energy) explains the cerebral caesuras, because in this way the water of the cerebrospinal fluid (CSF) can circulate quickly and deeply, reaching up to the neuron furthest from the ventricles and the subarachnoid space.

Although the discussion of water, so far, is largely focused on its properties as a solvent, it also serves as a ligand. For example, in both hemoglobin and cytochrome oxidase, the binding and subsequent release of water molecules is critical to their proper function and now in ahead with need to add a new possibility: water as substrate to energy production.

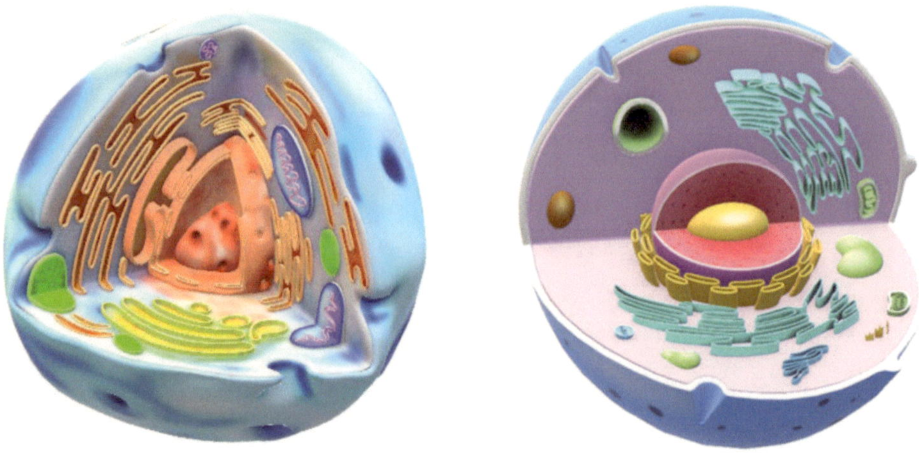

A B

Figure 5.
Melanin is usually not represented in the eukaryotic cell models available in the different sources of information.

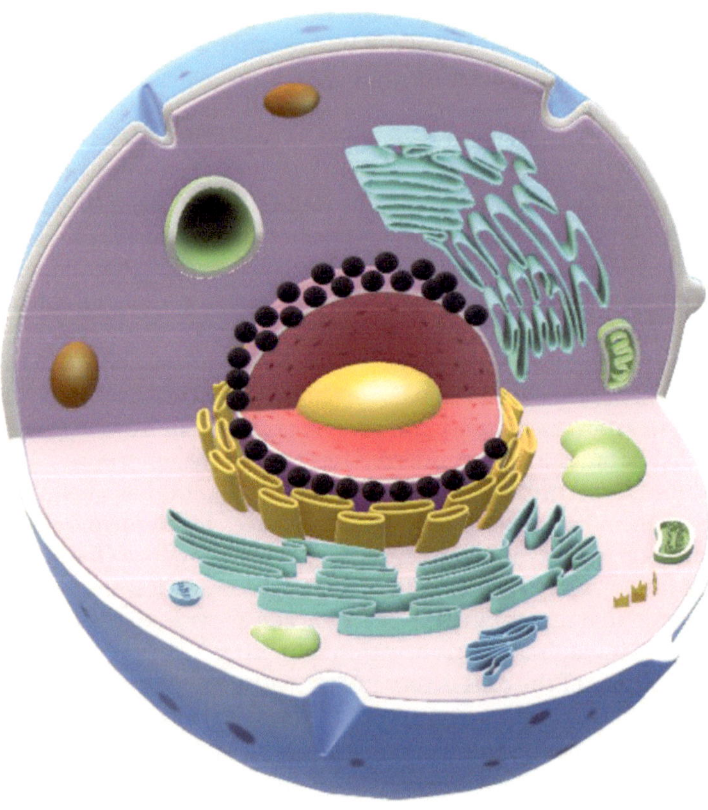

Figure 6.
Drawing of eukaryotic cell to which the melanosomes have been added in their most usual location, the perinuclear space, from releasing the energy symmetrically, in all directions, following the laws of simple diffusion. The melanosomes surround the cell nucleus, enveloping it in its entirety, thus constituting a constant source of energy for the largest intracellular organelle, since it contains neither mitochondria nor ATP.

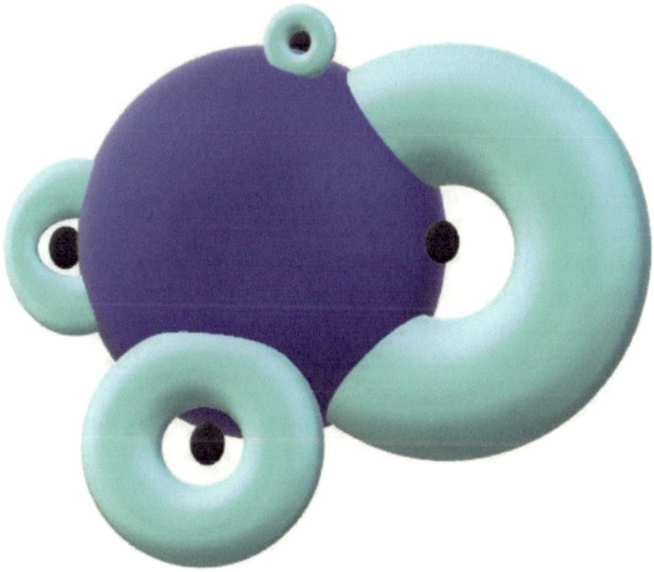

Figure 7.
Schematic representation of the cell nucleus (deep blue) and some melanosomes (black dots) of which emanate the growing spheres (light blue) composed of molecular hydrogen (H_2), which transports the energy that is released by dissociating the molecule of water. Molecular hydrogen easily crosses any membrane or barrier inside the cell, so the growing spheres provide energy to both the inside of the cell nucleus and the rest of the organelles located outer of the nucleus by inside cell membrane. That molecular hydrogen does not combine with water is a crucial physic-chemical of hydrogen characteristic that explains the normal displacement of molecular hydrogen (H_2) along cytoplasm.

The amount of chemical energy in the form of H_2 and high-energy electrons that eukaryotic cells need at any moment is surprisingly accurate, and when water or melanin physic-chemical properties are altered by pollution of the surroundings (pesticides, herbicides, fertilizers, metals, plastics, solvents, industrial waste, anesthetic agents, drugs, alcohol, variations in climate, cold, heat; etc.), the cell seems as it goes into imbalance, experiencing a turning-point in evolution.

1.4 The DNA code

It is a sequence of chemicals that form information that control how humans are made and how they work. It is a digital-like code, but it is not binary, but quaternary with four distinct items: adenosine (A), cytosine (C), guanine (G), and thymine (T).

These four substances are the fundamental "bits" of information in the genetic code and are called "base pairs" because there are actually two substances per "bit." Everything else is built on top of this basis of four DNA digits.

However, life origin cannot be explained arising from DNA. The sequence in melanin about dissociation and reformation of water, this is, liquid → gas → liquid → gas → liquid → gas, and so on, can be reduced to 0 (liquid) and 1 (gas), a kind of binary code and a binary code that gives origin and therefore also regulates a quaternary code has room to explain the origin and evolution of life.

The genetic code is not an autonomous system, as any other chemical process, nevertheless complicated, requires energy to be created, to replicate, to carry out their functions, and even to preserve the shape, because the water of the cytoplasm tend to separate the molecules.

The human genome is about 3 billion bases in total, and every human being has 2 copies of this code; one copy from each parent, thereby a human's cell DNA contains around 6 billion bases.

These 6 billion base pairs are split among 46 chromosomes. Each person gets 2 pairs of chromosomes, 23 from each parent, to total 46 chromosomes per human cell. A chromosome is the largest form of a DNA molecule, with a large sequence of DNA codes, of differing lengths, usually hundreds of millions of base pairs in each chromosome.

Chromosomes are independent molecules of DNA, with the typical double helix, a start and end, but no cycles. Each chromosome has subsequences of DNA bases that encode features, and these are called "genes." All genes have different lengths. The total number of distinct genes in the human genome is believed to be around 30,000 genes.

Most genes clearly encode the data sequence representing a specific protein that would be synthesized in the precise moment, right temporality, exact amount, and accurate location; therefore, a gene, besides constant energy supply, also requires detailed information to adequately carry out its highly complex functions. All the genes together are only a small part of DNA code. The 30,000 odd genes in human DNA might only make up 4% of human DNA.

The structure of DNA and RNA are very similar, but RNA uses uracil (U) instead of thymine (T). Proteins are a base-20 code using the 20 amino acids. DNA represents a protein that has an ordered sequence of base-4 triplets, using 64 possible values to 20 amino acids.

1.5 Genetic versus hereditary

The following phrase "Chronic Myeloid Leukemia (CLL) is a genetic disease, but not a hereditary disease" is confusing because in any disease some degree of altered gene expression can be expected. Therefore, most leukemia patients have no family history of the disease, and there is no evidence that it can be passed on to the children of someone living with the disease. Occasionally, there are families that may have other members living with leukemia, however, without taking in account the role of toxic compounds capable to perturb the generation and distribution of energy, never was and never will conclusive genetic evidence that family members are predisposed to develop leukemia.

There are diseases that are difficult to classify, i.e., the CLL that is a B-cell lymphoproliferative disorder and is one of the most common adult leukemias [20]. Although the cause remains unknown, a family history of the disease is one of the best characterized risk factors, but more for familial exposure to external toxic compounds than for theoretical minute punctual mutations or loci that cannot be found yet or even less to probe.

This is a long-lasting observation that is congruent with the fact that the genetic code is as perfect as everything else, instead what we see are groups of people (family members or factory workers) exposed to similar toxics.

The family groups share the same customs, the same food, the same house, the same trades or professions, the same environment, etc.

In fact, familial aggregation of the disease has been observed for decades, with multiple reports in the literature of families in whom the occurrence of CLL is greatly enriched with what appears to be almost Mendelian inheritance [21], and worst, there are environmental toxicants so persistent that can be transmitted from parents to child, for instance, through mother's milk.

"Along with its antibodies, enzymes and general goodness, breast milk also contains dozens of compounds that have been linked to negative health effects," bisphenol A (BPA, a plastic component), PBDEs (used in flame retardants), perchlorate (used in rocket fuel), perfluorinated chemicals (PFCs, used in floor cleaners and nonstick pans), phthalates (used in plastics), polyvinyl chloride (PVC, commonly known as vinyl), organochlorine pesticides, dioxin, benzene (a known human carcinogen [22]), and the heavy metals cadmium, lead, and mercury as leading offenders [23].

Risk of childhood leukemia is increased for benzene exposures of > 10 μg/m^3 associated with traffic [24] and auto repair garages and gasoline stations [25].

Human milk serves as a valuable biological matrix for the assessment of public and environmental health. The more lipophilic the chemical is, the more likely it is to be found in human milk. By the way, the bone marrow has a high content of lipids.

Family predisposition should be understood as epigenetic predisposition, as external factors such as contaminated air, contaminated water, polluted air, contaminated food, pesticides, herbicides, fertilizers, metals, plastics, solvents, industrial waste, shocks, addiction drugs, emotional strains, etc.

Such factors are common to the group of people we define as family; these are father, mother, siblings, and sometimes close relatives who live in the same house.

The exposure to exogenous factors in factory employees is called professional risk, as is the newly sounded case of leukemia in Samsung employees. And the difference between one and another example is only the name that we put, because both in the families and in the factories, the effect of the toxins is similar as they alter the delicate balance between mass and energy in the processes that make up the life, in this case in the complex functions of the bone marrow.

Familial CLL does not appear to differ from sporadic CLL in terms of prognostic markers and clinical outcome [26].

But such external factors only modify the genetic expression in one way or another, but they do not have an effect that we could call direct on the DNA chains or their components. In fact, what is importantly affected is the generation and distribution of energy that emanates from melanin, and hence, general failures, characteristic of disturbances in the generation, and distribution of energy begin to happen, as it happens in any system.

So, it is to date, the identification of genes that predisposes to chronic familial leukemia has been unsuccessful in real terms, which is attributed to various factors, such as the small number of affected individuals susceptible to being studied and technological limitations or maybe because there are many genes affected and each contributes a little [27].

Farming-related exposure and occupational chemicals increase risk of CLL. This is congruent with population-based studies and cohorts that have shown significant family aggregation in CLL and related conditions such as non-Hodgkin lymphoma and other lymphomas; and on the other hand, the absolute risk of a first-degree family member for the development of CLL or a similar disease is very low.

Thereby, linkage studies have been conducted in high-risk CLL families to screen the whole genome for loci that contribute to susceptibility, but no gene mutations have yet been identified by this method.

The accumulation of small, mature-appearing lymphocytes in the bone marrow, blood, and lymphoid tissues in CLL indicates that many germ cells are altered, as well as the daughter cells that are produced. The possibilities that a point mutation (loci) or the joint failure of several genes occurs in a significant portion of the germ cells and that such dysfunction is also expressed in the daughter cells is so unlikely that it has not been able to prove much least explain.

On the contrary, a failure in the generation and distribution of energy from melanin that is repeated in numerous cells both germs and daughters is so feasible that it can easily be demonstrated, as is the case of the experiment described in Section 2.4.

Incidence rates in men are nearly twice as high as in women that can be explained due to men are exposed to environmental toxics more often than women. Although advanced age, white ancestry (less melanin equal to less water dissociation) and family history of hematologic malignancies are risk factors; the etiology of CLL is still not understood more than unknown [28].

1.6 Energy failure means generalized dysfunction: arsenic poisoning

In any system, when the failure is widespread, energy is the usual or main cause. And in the case of the eukaryotic cell, alterations are diffuse, so they can be found at any level, including genes, histones, chromosomes, etc. The study of cellular structures separately from the flow of energy leads to biased conclusions, because the mass and the energy are inseparable in the real world.

Any structural alteration of the cell is preceded and accompanied by a disturbance in the flow of energy that comes from the dissociation of the water, which happens inside the melanin. The name of the affected structures or substances (protein, histone, amino acid, nucleotide, gene, chromosome, etc.), does not have more relevance, because the cell ignores it; there is simply an imbalance between mass and energy.

The cell uses the energy in many ways, and it does in a surprisingly exact way, leaving almost nothing at random; as it has done since the beginning of time. When the amount of chemical energy available in the form of molecular hydrogen (H_2) and high-energy electrons(*e*-) is not enough to fill the energy needs of the cell, then the role of chance begins to be significant, so the clinical manifestations also depend on chance, but the basic problem is still the same: balance between mass and energy.

1.7 Leukemia, a generalized failure?

Leukemia is cancer that starts in the tissue that forms blood. Most blood cells develop from cells in the bone marrow called stem cells. In a person with leukemia, the bone marrow makes abnormal white blood cells. The abnormal cells are leukemia cells. Unlike normal blood cells, leukemia cells do not die when they should. These may crowd out abnormal white blood cells, red blood cells, and platelets. This makes it hard for normal blood cells to do their work. The four main types of leukemias are acute lymphoblastic leukemia (ALL), acute myelogenous leukemia (AML), chronic lymphocytic leukemia (CLL), and chronic myelogenous leukemia (CML).

The risk factors already described in leukemia are genetic disorders, radiation exposure, physical and chemical exposures, and chemotherapy.

The greater incidence of leukemia per 100,000 persons is in white races, with 17.5/10.7 (male/female), and in black race, the incidence per 100,000 persons is 12.9/8.0, suggesting that a greater amount of melanin in the skin or body is a protective factor.

Supposedly, a clone of invasive cells may arise at any stage of cell maturation and specialization in the lymphoid, myeloid, or pluripotential stage. The cause of this apparent clonal development is quite unknown in most cases; it appears to involve the rearrangement of sequence of bases on DNA molecules or chromosomal instability syndrome.

External and internal factors such as ionizing radiation and chemicals favor chromosomal anomalies. These random DNA changes will lead to an uncontrollable mitosis of cells.

These leukemic blasts show abnormal behavior infiltrating into the bone marrow, altering, by means of diverse mechanisms, the astonishing accuracies of the normal processes of hematopoiesis (formation of cellular components of blood).

The abnormal cells eventually infiltrate into other organs as such as the spleen, the eye, or the liver, also disrupting the astonishing accuracy of their regular processes.

The blood becomes unable to carry out its functions, and the individual affected will experience within a few days or weeks increased fatigue and infections and will bruise and bleed more easily than they usually would have.

The clinical findings of leukemia, such as thrombocytopenia, anemia, severe infections widespread, bone pain, arthralgias, and involvement of the liver, spleen, thymus, lymph nodes, skin, gums, eye, head (CNS), and neck; it is compatible with a generalized system failure, which is typical of problems in the generation and distribution of energy (from light/melanin/water).

The experiment that we describe below points in that direction (**Figures 8–28**).

1.8 Arsenic (As)

It is a metalloid with atomic number 33, atomic mass of 74.92, and oxidation number: ± 3, 5. It alters multiple metabolic pathways by supposedly uncoupling oxidative phosphorylation. Its effect is not specific; it attacks several organs and is tasteless and odorless. The ingestion of arsenic induces a general failure of the organism, suggesting that arsenic acts by disturbing the amazingly accurate generation and distribution of energy.

Arsenic binds the cofactor sulfhydryl, dihydrolipoate, which inhibits the oxidative metabolic pathway of pyruvate and succinate. The body also replaces arsenic with phosphorus, which inhibits oxidative phosphorylation, but the most significant alteration seems to be the inhibition of sulfhydryl.

Arsenic pentavalent is well absorbed by the GI tract, and it is initially located in blood, coupled with globulin; thereafter, redistribution occurs within following 24 hours mainly to the liver, lungs, intestine, and spleen. Arsenic replaces the phosphorus of the bone, where it remains 30 years or more.

Arsenic, when decoupling the oxidative phosphorylation, induces a significant decrease in the availability of energy of the cell. However, arsenic affects the melanin itself, because they have great affinity with each other, so arsenic (As) not

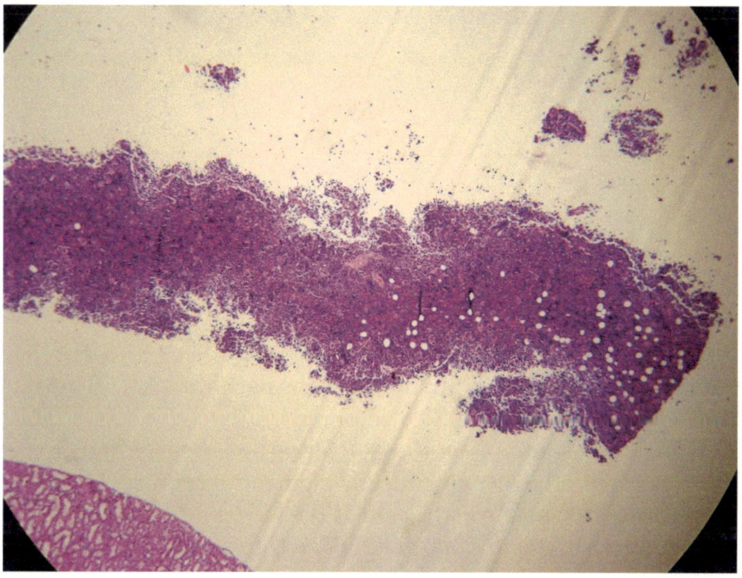

Figure 8.
Bone marrow, control group (A), H&E, 5X.

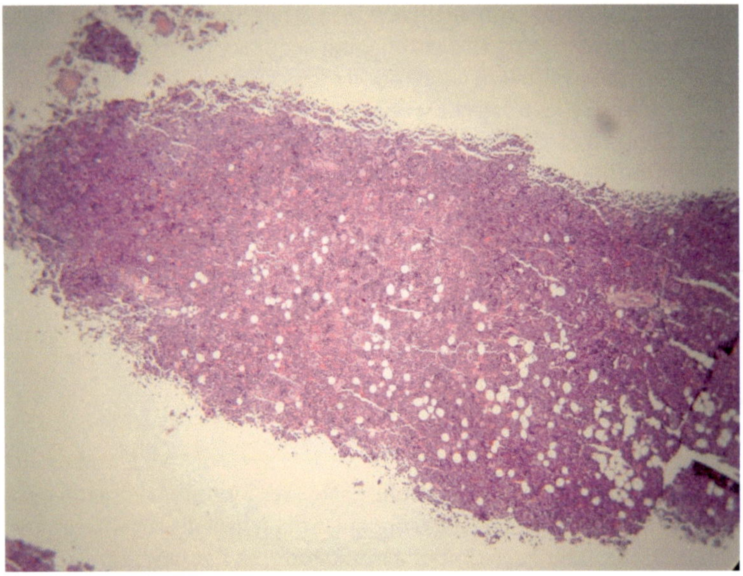

Figure 9.
Bone marrow, exposed group (B) to arsenic. H&E, 5X.

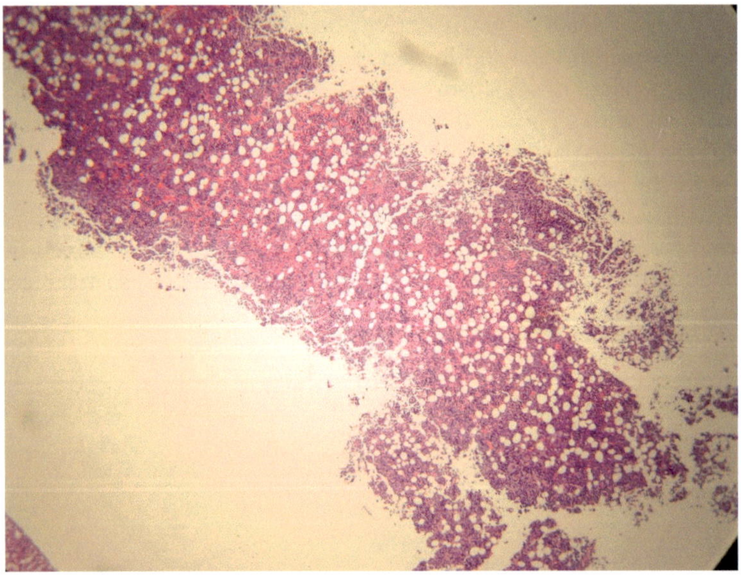

Figure 10.
Bone marrow. Group C exposed to arsenic and treated at the same time. H&E, 5X.

only damages the complex energy distribution system arising from the dissociation of the water molecule by melanin but damages the melanin itself, disturbing the generation of energy, so the damage is widespread.

Arsenic in small doses stimulates the generation and distribution of energy from melanin, so it is, in the seventeenth and eighteenth century, was used by the aristocracy in France to rejuvenate the skin of the face.

Furthermore, in the fifteenth century, William Withering, who discovered digitalis, was a strong proponent of arsenic-based therapies [29]. He argued, "Poisons in small doses are the best medicines; and the best medicines in too large doses are poisonous".

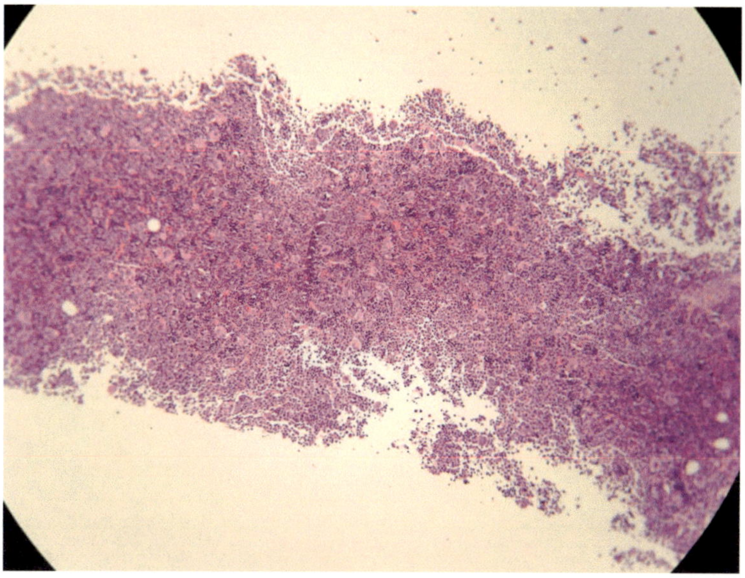

Figure 11.
Bone marrow, control group (A). H&E, 10X.

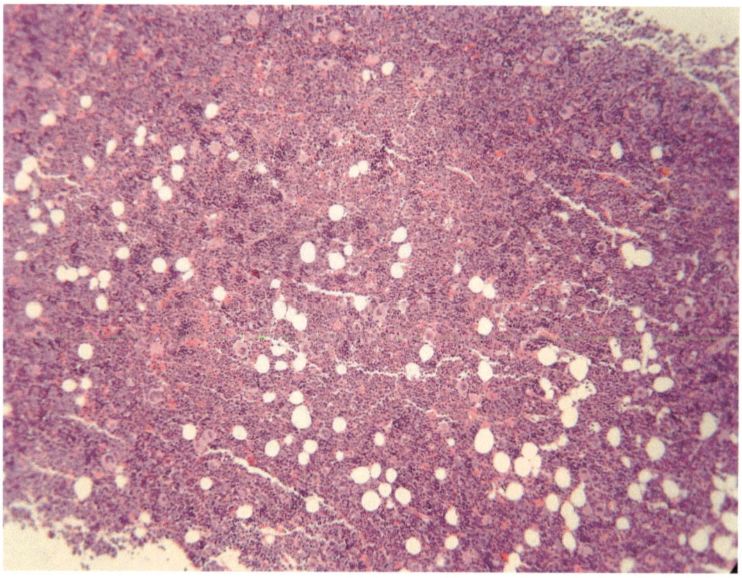

Figure 12.
Bone marrow. Exposed group (B) to arsenic in water. H&E, 10X.

Thomas Fowler compounded a potassium bicarbonate-based solution of arsenic trioxide (As_2O_3) and was used empirically to treat a variety of diseases during the eighteenth, nineteenth, and early twentieth centuries [30]. In 1910, Nobel Laureate and Paul Ehrlich developed Salvarsan, an organic arsenical for treating syphilis and trypanosomiasis.

But in higher doses, the opposite effect occurs; therefore, chronic exposure is a serious with arsenic public health problem in some parts of the world [31]. Intoxication by this heavy metal can result from breathing sawdust, workplace air, or arsenic-preserved wood or from ingesting contaminated water, food, or soil [32].

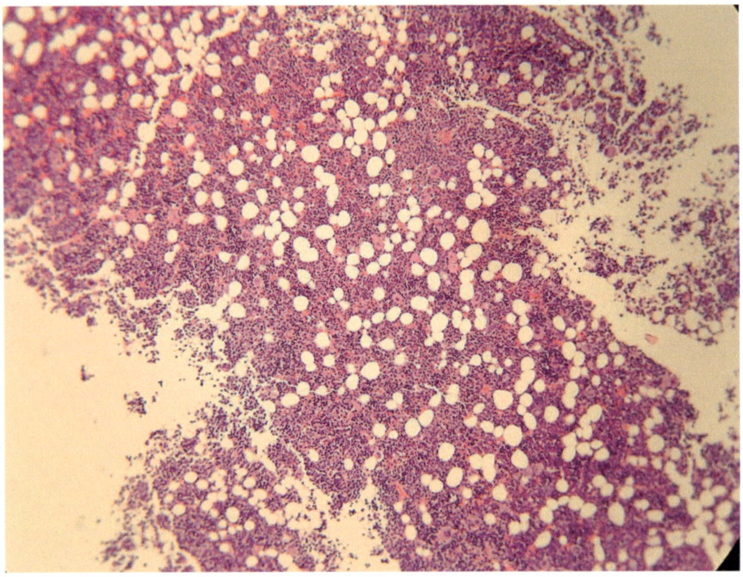

Figure 13.
Bone marrow. Group C exposed to arsenic in water and treated at the same time. H&E, 10X.

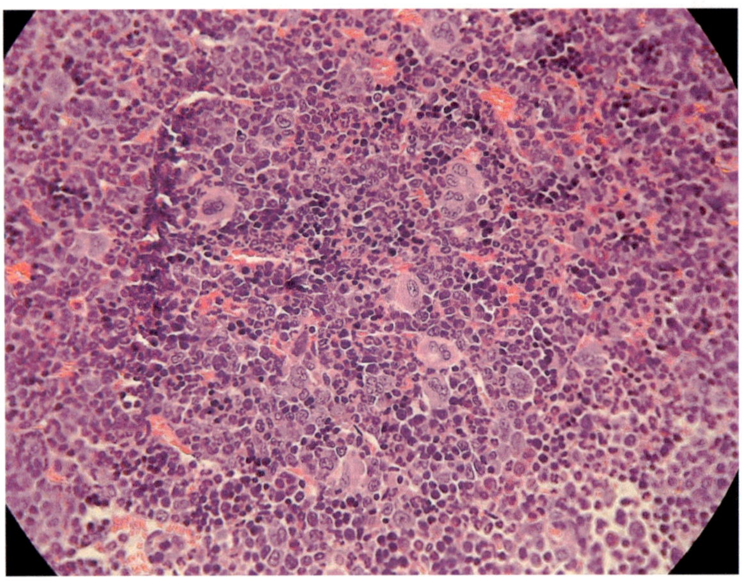

Figure 14.
Bone marrow, control group (A). H&E, 40X.

Contamination of groundwater happens by naturally occurring arsenic, also by widespread use of arsenic-containing herbicides and pesticides; its incorporation into feed as a substance to promote the growth of livestock and poultry and its industrial use has caused the environmental arsenic dispersion.

Biomagnification of arsenic is observed in many species of fish and shellfish. Sadly, the average daily human intake of arsenic is approximately 300 μg, mainly ingested with food and water. The World Health Organization (WHO) safe limit for arsenic in drinking water is 0.01 mg/L.

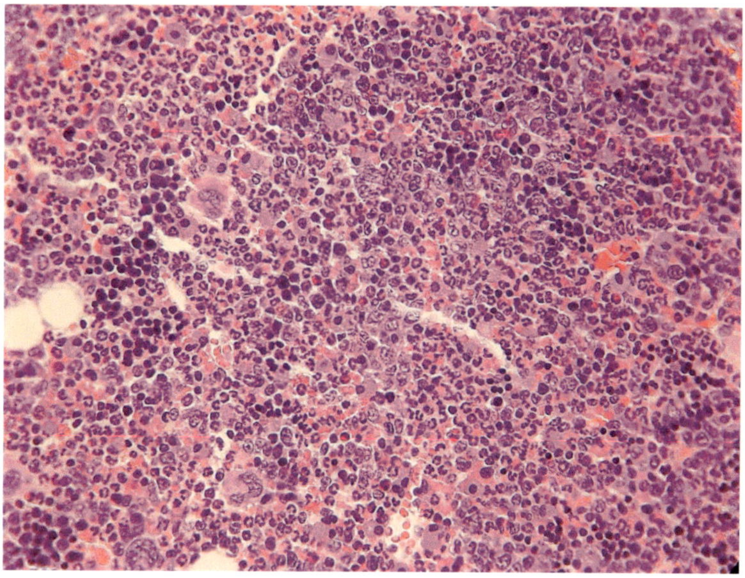

Figure 15.
Bone marrow. Exposed group (B) to arsenic in water. H&E, 40X.

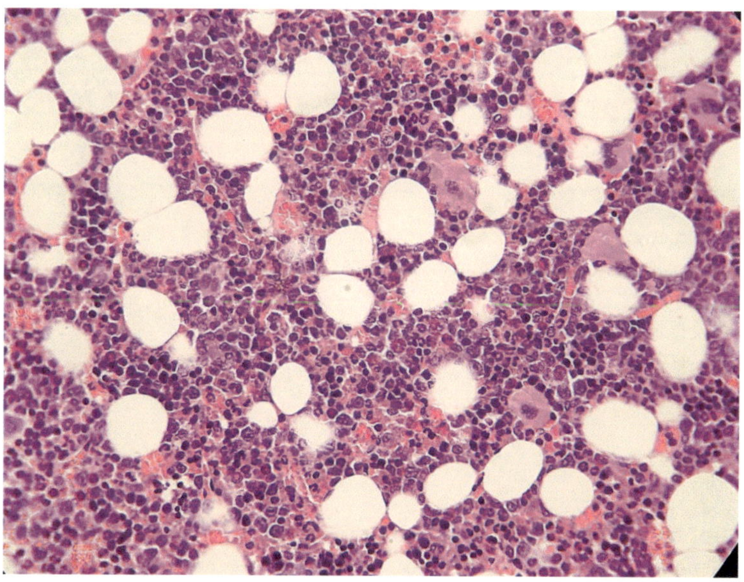

Figure 16.
Bone marrow. Group C exposed to arsenic in water and treated at the same time. H&E, 40X.

Acute and chronic poisoning of arsenic can be confused with hemorrhagic gastroenteritis, cardiac arrhythmias, and psychiatric disease. In 1878, Boston City Hospital described the effect of Fowler's solution on the reduction of white blood cells in two normal people and one patient with "leukocythemia" [33].

Subsequently, As_2O_3 was administered as a primary antileukemic agent until it was replaced by radiation therapy. In 1930, the hematologic use of arsenic experienced a resurgence in popularity, when its efficacy was reported in patients with chronic myelogenous leukemia [34].

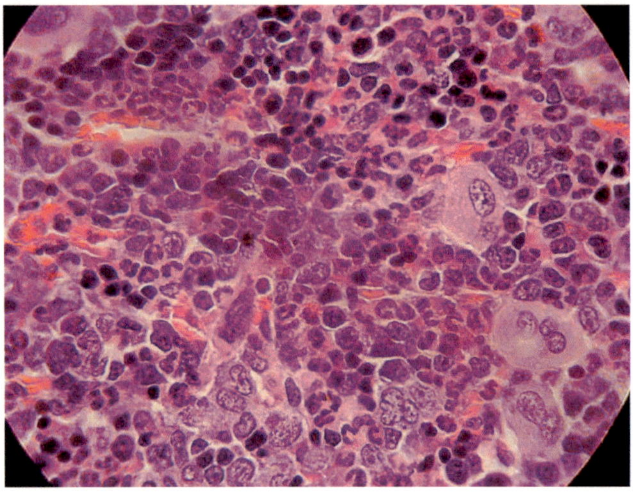

Figure 17.
Bone marrow. Control group A. H&E, 100 X.

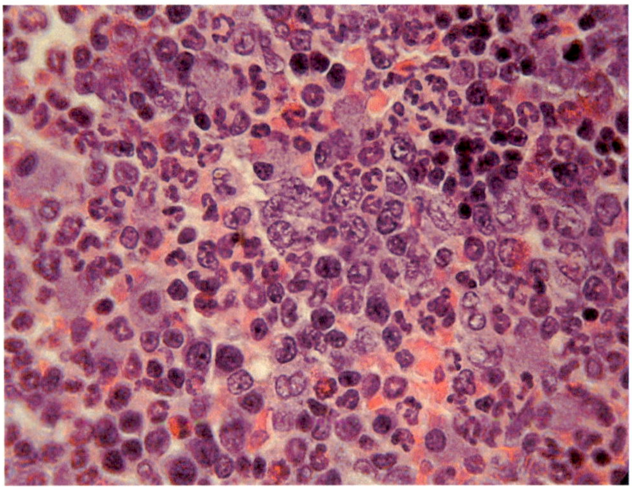

Figure 18.
Bone marrow. Group B exposed to arsenic in water. H&E, 100X.

Until supplanted by modern chemotherapy, arsenic trioxide after radiation was considered the most effective treatment for CML and other types of leukemia. Recently, reports from China have described the induction of clinical and hematological responses by arsenic trioxide in patients with de novo and relapsed acute promyelocytic leukemia (APL) [35]. This is an important observation, since around 20–30% of patients with this form of acute myelogenous leukemia relapse despite treatment with all-trans retinoic acid and combination chemotherapy.

Arsenic treatment was not associated with bone marrow suppression and produced only limited side effects. Thereby, arsenic trioxide (Trisenox®) was approved for the treatment of relapsed or refractory APL by the US Food and Drug Administration in September 2000.

It is interesting that the therapeutic application of arsenic in low dose is widely used. Due to generalized systemic effects, so far, a clear explanation about its therapeutic effects is not available. It is possible that other similar therapies, based in toxic compounds as all-trans retinoic acid and daunorubicin/doxorubicin/

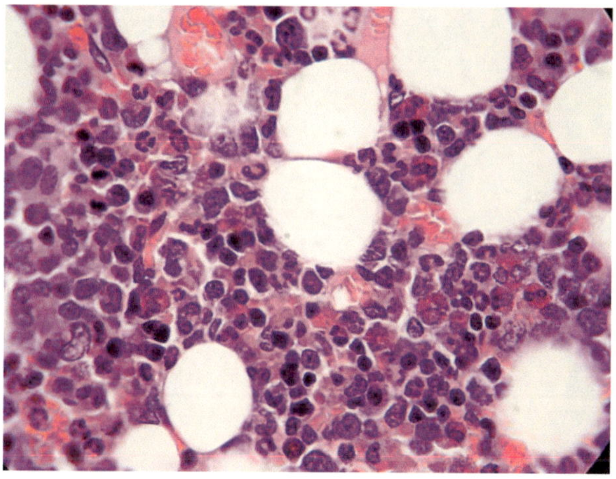

Figure 19.
Bone marrow. Group C exposed to arsenic in water and treated at the same time. H&E, 100X.

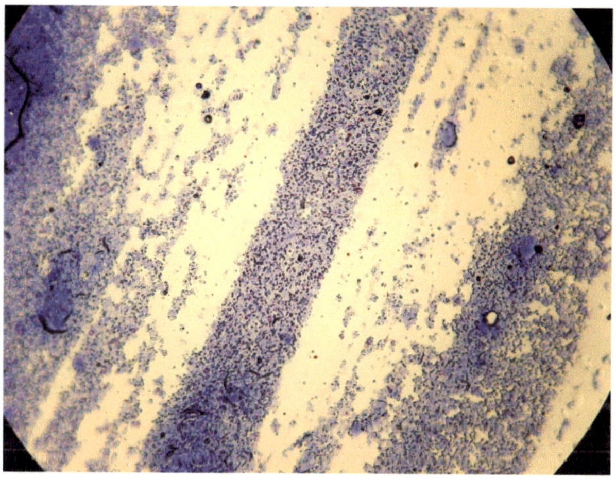

Figure 20.
Peripheral blood smear. Control group A. Giemsa stain. 10X.

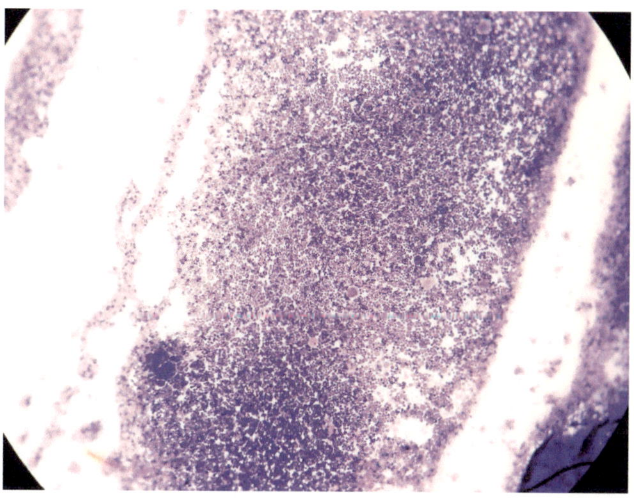

Figure 21.
Peripheral blood smear. Group B exposed to arsenic in water. Giemsa stain, 10X.

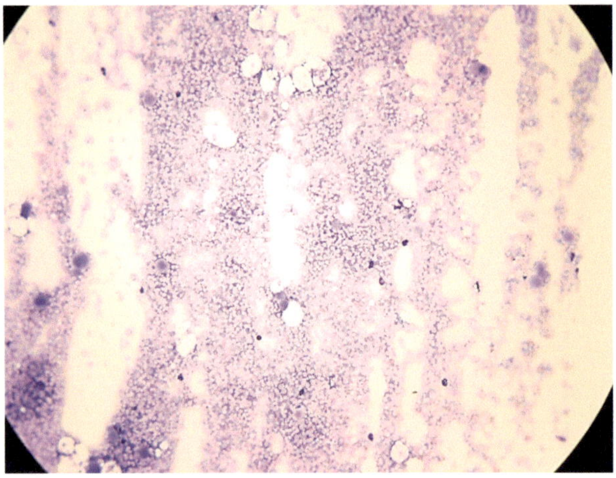

Figure 22.
Peripheral blood smear. Group C exposed to arsenic in water and treated at the same time. Giemsa stain, 10X.

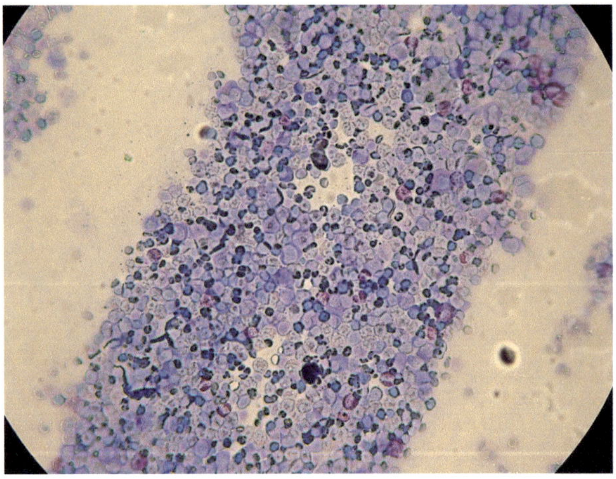

Figure 23.
Peripheral blood smear. Control group A. Giemsa stain, 40X.

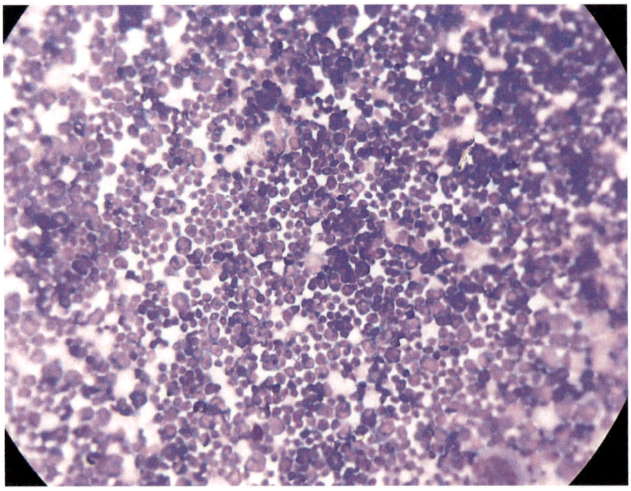

Figure 24.
Peripheral blood smear. Group B exposed to arsenic in water. Giemsa stain, 40X.

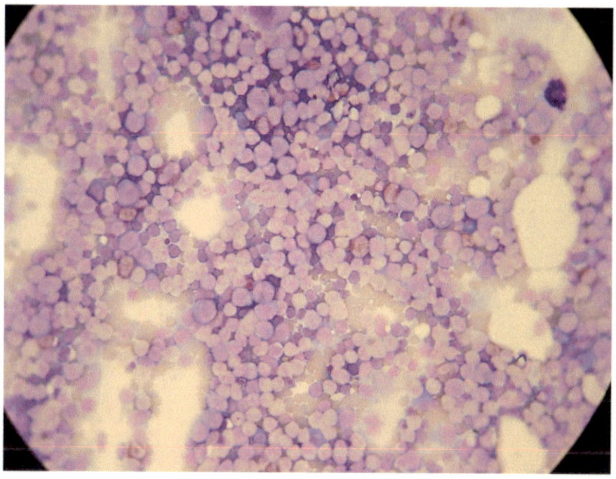

Figure 25.
Peripheral blood smear. Group C exposed to arsenic in water and treated at the same time. Giemsa stain, 40X.

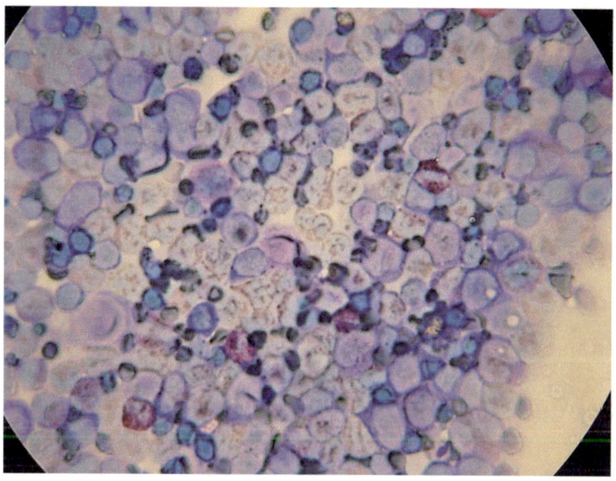

Figure 26.
Peripheral blood smear. Control group A. Giemsa stain, 100X.

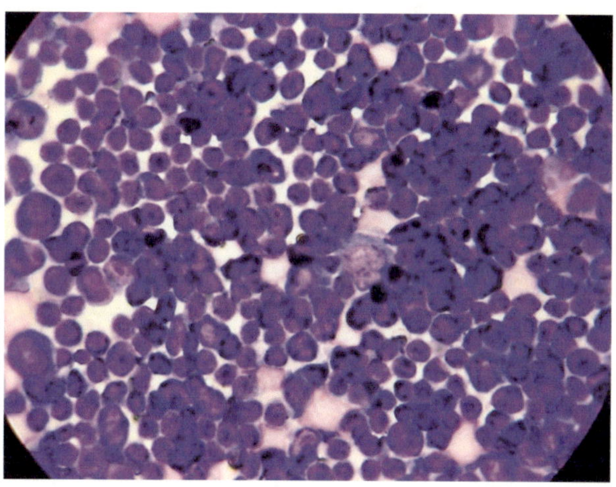

Figure 27.
Peripheral blood smear. Group B exposed to arsenic in water. Giemsa stain, 100X.

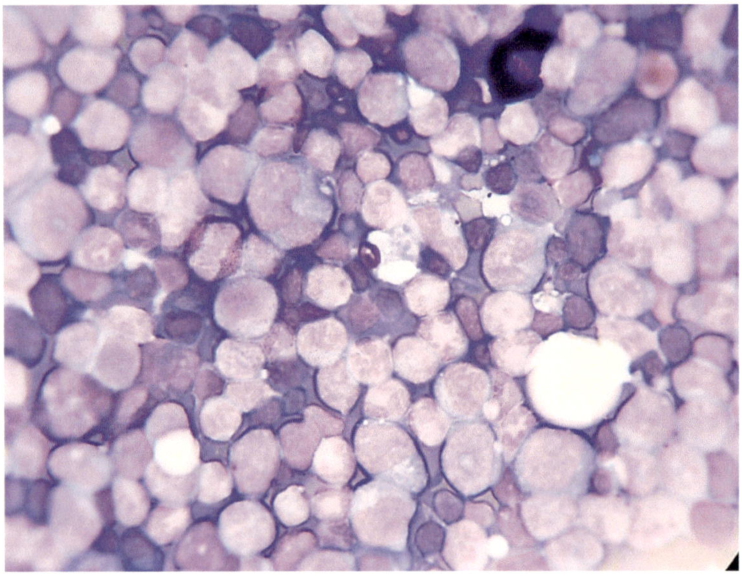

Figure 28.
Peripheral blood smear. Group C exposed to arsenic in water and treated at the same time. Giemsa stain, 100X.

epirubicin/idarubicin, an anthracycline-related compounds [36], are altering gene expression (genotoxic agents) through different pathways; thereby their effect is generalized, so it can be expected that it also affects the generation and flow of energy from melanin.

Arsenic, all trans-retinoic acid, and anthracycline-related compounds, when it is used at very high doses, then the amazingly accurate process of generation and distribution of energy, from the dissociation of the water molecule by melanin, stops almost completely, so death occurs in minutes.

Therefore, the administration of arsenic in laboratory animals is an easy way to induce general dysfunction or failure, as we are altering a fundamental process of life as is the generation and distribution of melanin energy.

Our working hypothesis was to induce widespread failure in rats and to study the effects on different tissues, such as the lung, kidney, liver, etc. [37]. The results in kidney and liver were published already. This is the first publication of results in the bone marrow.

2. Materials and methods

There were 3 groups of 10 Wistar rats each one, all males, adults. Group A was control. Group B was the exposed group to arsenic in water. The administration of pentavalent arsenic was 0.50 mg/L in the water and administered ad libitum. Group C was the group exposed to arsenic in the same way as group B and treated at the same time with a novel formula that restores the balance between mass and energy.

3. Results

The results of the experiment were according to what was expected. The administration of pentavalent arsenic was 0.50 mg/L in the water. Arsenic is a toxic and a carcinogen; among the noncarcinogenic harmful effects of this metalloid, the most common associated with its ingestion are those presented in the skin, hyperpigmentation, agent hypopigmentation, and hyperkeratosis, damage to the cardiovascular system; renal and hepatic alterations, development of peripheral neuropathies and encephalopathies; and its capacity of endocrine disruptor related to the development of diabetes. The relationship between the presence of arsenic in water in several regions and the increase in the presence and mortality of the bladder, lung, kidney, and hepatic cancer has been recognized in the potentially exposed populations.

As described in literature and as we observed in the histological slides of the group of animals exposed to arsenic (group B), the damage is generalized. It would be necessary to elaborate multiple conjectures to try to explain the diffuse impairment to organs and systems that are produced from the ingestion of arsenic in the water. However, the significant disturbance caused by arsenic in the generation and distribution of energy derived from melanin, it could explain the different levels of microscopic alterations observed in the histological stains of the lung, kidney, liver, spleen, bone marrow, etc.

According to the adage that good experiments are those with few animals, many results are obtained; group B was constituted with only ten animals, and the size of the effect of arsenic was substantive. On the other hand, it fulfilled the observed fact that in any system, when the fault is widespread, we must think first of energy.

So, we can think that, in this experiment, we could induce and thereby demonstrated in a reasonable way that the widespread failure caused by arsenic ingestion is due to the perturbations of the generation and distribution of energy derived from melanin.

The findings of group C—exposed and treated at the same time—cast better than expected findings, because on the one hand, the generalized toxicity of arsenic manifested itself again, but significantly decreased by the simultaneous administration of the therapeutic drug. And on the other hand, we could demonstrate the usefulness of our therapy to prevent and treat the general failure of organs and systems that is induced with the ingestion of arsenic that also gives a real hope for the many patients in similar situation.

The improvement with the treatment was also manifested in the different tissues studied, which is consistent with the fact that, by reducing the alteration in the generation and distribution of energy, the improvement is detectable at the microscopic level and it is also a general improvement.

The induced changes during the experiment with the exposure and treatment mean widespread effects, positive and negatives. The size of the effect is noticeable in both cases, exposure and treatment. And the magnitude of the effect was similar in other tissues in which biopsy was taken.

The observable findings under the microscope are very interesting, as they involve numerous variables such as cell size, shape, color changes, etc. But there are so many changes that are hard to explain based only in analysis of observable structures.

The improvement in group C (treated and exposed) is notorious. Thereby, two hypotheses were tested with one experiment, few animals, and many results, a good experiment. The way melanin releases energy, symmetrically and in all directions, in the manner of growing spheres that follow the laws of simple diffusion, flooding of molecular hydrogen cytosol, allows the vast majority of chemical reactions to be driven by these hydrogen molecules, which are not combined with water, so they only move through it reaching until the last corner of the eukaryotic cells with its precious energy charge and its powerful antioxidant effect.

Therefore, when the generation and distribution of energy that comes from melanin is altered or at least disturbed by environmental factors, of a chemical or physical nature, many biochemical processes are randomly affected by the decrease in energy levels.

We must not forget that intracellular biochemical processes are surprisingly accurate in every one of their physical and chemical characteristics, as they have been since the beginning of time. But the exact chemical reactions require in turn to be driven by an exact amount of energy. And only a molecule as wonderful as melanin has the necessary bioenergetic capacity.

The multiple tissue changes observable in the histological images of the rat and arsenic experiment underpin the concept of the unsuspected bioenergetic role of melanin. The structural changes susceptible to being observed in the light microscope and stains Giemsa, in the case of the smears, and hematoxylin and eosin, in the case of histological cuts, allow to glimpse that the number of factors involved is vast.

And analyzing one by one from a structural point of view, without considering the incessant flow of energy, would lead us to the same errors that we currently observe in the literature. It is a fact that the cell uses energy in many ways, and in studying cell biology, we must be aware that even to study ultrastructure alone, our technological resources are relatively limited.

4. Discussion

The changes that we observed in the experiment are very interesting and highly significant, it would be very difficult to explain them based on genes, since genes are not autonomous, because they depend on the energy and surrounding cell scaffolding to replicate, express themselves and even to preserve the form, stability and function. They are also immersed in a highly complex biological system, with which they interact in a way that is not yet understood, but all the components of this highly complex system depend entirely on the energy that emanates from the melanin, so that by restoring the generation and Energy distribution, which it is so fundamental, then it is possible to explain the positive and negative changes that we could observe under the light microscope.

Characteristically, energy failures produce widespread alterations, we can say otherwise, when the problem of energy is improved or corrected, then many processes are in turn restored, which can be detected by microscopically examining the cellular structure, which is all what we can value, being an indirect indicator of the flow of energy.

Simplistically, if the ultrastructure is altered, the generation and distribution of energy is indeed disturbed, in a directly proportional form, and vice versa. That is why, despite many efforts, trying to explain diseases such as leukemia, based on purely observations of the structure, for example genes, histones or chromosomes, has given so far poor results, it is necessary to consider at the same time the highly dynamic generation and distribution of energy.

5. Conclusion

The current medicine is ensnared in the dogma that a single molecule, glucose, provides energy and mass at the same time; furthermore it also considers that only the chlorophyll of plants can transform the luminous energy into chemical energy by means of the dissociation of the water molecule. On the other hand, analyzing in a separate way the microstructure (mass) and the energy flow in the cells has led to important biases since the mass and energy are inseparable in the real world.

Trying to find the cause or explanation of diseases, based merely on the study of observable of micro or ultrastructural alterations has produced very limited results, because the cell is a highly dynamic living entity, in which the flow of energy and mass are incessant and inseparable. The optimal thing would be to study both phenomena (mass and energy) at the same time and in real time, which is not currently feasible.

During the study of biological phenomena, we must keep in mind that the size of the effect should be large [38]; otherwise, when the size of the effect is small, we end up studying in detail some prevalent bias. Bias is defined as the combination of various design, data, analysis, and presentation factors that tend to produce research findings when they should not be produced. There is an increasing concern that most current published research findings are false. The extremely large studies may be more likely to find a formally statistically significant difference for a trivial effect that is not meaningfully different from the null hypothesis [39].

It is likely that current unawareness of physicians about the human body's ability to take light energy and the impoverishment of it by environment toxicants is a significant factor of the poor performance of health systems. For instance, in the USA, 225000 annual deaths are estimated due to unnecessary surgeries, errors in patient medication, errors of different types in hospitals; nosocomial infections, and adverse effects of medications [40]. Most of the data are derived from studies in hospitalized patients, thereby are estimates of death only and do not include adverse effects associated with disability or discomfort.

Therefore between 4% and 18% experience adverse effects in outpatient settings, with 116 million extra physician visits, 8 million hospitalizations, 3 million long-term admissions, 199.000 additional deaths, and $77 billion in extra costs [41].

The specific alterations of the genes cannot explain the diseases called genetic or hereditary, because the influence of genes is relatively limited and highly complex, i.e., the cystic fibrosis gene, codify to almost 600 proteins. Furthermore, disturbances in the generation and distribution of energy from melanin can manifest—structurally—as alterations in the genes, since the replication and the expression of chromosomes require an astonishing accurate source and level of available energy in the form of molecular hydrogen (H_2) and high-energy electrons (*e*-).

And if we consider the effects of energy flow not only in the cell nucleus, histones, genes, and chromosomes but also in the scaffolding around them, things become even more incomprehensible to us; but to have understood that the energy of the cell comes from the light-melanin-water triad in order of abundance in the universe, and that it does not come from glucose, represents a critical advance in the knowledge, which can be translated in an expedited way to the clinic, for the benefit of the patient, especially if we take into account the role of environmental toxins and their detrimental and generalized effects on the amazingly accurate process of generation and distribution of energy by melanin.

Acknowledgements

This work was supported by Human Photosynthesis® Research Center, Aguascalientes 2000, México.

Author details

Arturo Solis Herrera
Human Photosynthesis® Research Center, Aguascalientes, México

*Address all correspondence to: comagua2000@yahoo.com

References

[1] Van Schaeybroeck S, Johnston PG. Abeloff's Clinical Oncology. Fifth ed. Churchill Livingstone; 2014. ISBN 978-1-4557-2865-7

[2] Nicholson JM, Cimini D. Chapter seven: Link between aneuploidy and chromosome instability. International Review of Cell and Molecular Biology. 2015;**315**:299-317. DOI: 10.1016/bs.ircmb 2014.11.002

[3] Mariño-Ramirez L, Kann MG, Shoemaker BA, Landsman D. Histone structure and nucleosome stability. Expert Review of Proteomics. 2005;**2**(5):719-729

[4] Ladurner AG. Inactivating chromosomes a macro domain that minimizes transcription. Molecular Cell. 2003;**12**(1):1-3

[5] Peterson CL, Laniel MA. Histories and histone modifications. Current Biology. 2004;**14**(14):R546-R551

[6] Lengauer C, Kinzler KW, Vogelstein B. Genetic instability in colorectal cancers. Nature. 1997;**386**:623-627

[7] Geigl JB, Obenauf AC, Schwarzbraun T, Speicher MR. Defining "chromosomal instability". Trends in Genetics. 2008;(2):64-69. DOI: 10.1016/j.tig 2007.11.006

[8] Michor F, Iwasa Y, Vogelstein B, Lengauer C, Nowak MA. Can chromosomal instability initiate tumorigenesis? Seminars in Cancer Biology. 2005;**15**(1):43-49

[9] Michor F, Iwasa Y, Rajagopalan H, Lengauer C, Nowak MA. Linear model of colon cancer initiation. Cell Cycle. 2004;**3**(3):358-362

[10] Komarova N. Does cancer solve an optimization problem? Cell Cycle. 2004;**3**(7):840-844

[11] Woo RA, Poon RY. Cell Cycle. Cyclin-dependent kinases and S phase control in mammalian cells. 2004;**3**(9):1101-1103

[12] Rankin EB, Narla A, Park J, Lin S, Sakamoto KM. Biology of the bone marrow microenvironment and myelodysplastic syndromes. Molecular Genetics and Metabolism. 2015;**116**(0):24-28. DOI: 10.1016/j. ymgme.2015.07.004

[13] Bianco P, Riminucci M, Robey PG. Bone marrow stromal stem cells: Nature, biology, and potential applications. Stem Cells. 2001;**19**(3):180-192

[14] Spencer JA, Ferraro F, Roussakis E, Klein A, Wu J, Runnels JM, et al. Direct measurement of local oxygen concentration in the bone marrow of live animals. Nature. 2014;**508**(7495):269-273

[15] Kresge N, Simoni RD, Hill RL. Otto Fritz Meyerhof and the elucidation of the glycolytic pathway. The Journal of Biological Chemistry. 2005;**280**:c3

[16] Kornberg H. Krebs and his trinity of cycles. Nature Reviews. Molecular Cell Biology. 2000;**1**:225-228

[17] Mitchell P. Coupling of phosphorylation to electron and hydrogen transfer by a chemi-osmotic type of mechanism. Nature. 1961;**191**:144-148

[18] Solis-Herrera A, Arias-Esparza MC, Ashraf GMC, Zamyatnin A Jr, Gjumrakch A. Beyond mitochondria, what would be the energy source of the cell? Central Nervous System Agents in Medicinal Chemistry. 2015;**15**:32-41

[19] Fiordaliso F, Leri A, Cesselli D, Limana F, Safai B, Nadal-Ginard B, et al. Hyperglycemia activates p53

and p53-regulated genes leading to myocyte cell death. Diabetes. 2001;**50**:2363-2375

[20] Brown JR. Inherited predisposition to chronic lymphocytic leukemia. Expert Review of Hematology. 2008;**1**(1):51-61. DOI: 10.1586/17474086.1.1.51

[21] Sellick GS, Catovsky D, Houlston RS. Familial chronic lymphocytic leukemia. Seminars in Oncology. 2006;**33**(2):195-201

[22] WHO IARC. IARC Monographs on the Evaluation of the Carcinogenic Risk of Chemicals to Humans 1987 (Suppl. 7)

[23] Kim SR, Halden RU, Buckley TJ. Volatile organic compounds in human Milk: Methods and measurements. Environmental Science & Technology. 2007;**41**(5):1662-1667. DOI: 10.1021/es062362y Publication Date (Web): February 1, 2007

[24] Crosignani P, Tittarelli A, Borgini A, Codazzi T, Rovelli A, Porro E, et al. Childhood leukemia and road traffic: A population-based case-control study. International Journal of Cancer. 2004;**108**:596-599

[25] Steffen C, Auclerc MF, Auvrignon A, Baruchel A, Kebaili K, Lambilliotte A, et al. Acute childhood leukaemia and environmental exposure to potential sources of benzene and other hydrocarbons; a case-control study. Occupational and Environmental Medicine. 2004;**61**:773-778

[26] Goldin RL, Landgren O, Marti GE, Caporaso NE. Familial aspects of chronic lymphocytic Leukemia, monoclonal B-cell lymphocytosis (MBL), and related lymphomas. European journal of Clinical and Medical Oncology. 2010;**2**(1):119-126

[27] Slager SL, Kay NE, Fredericksen ZS, et al. Susceptibility genes and B-chronic lymphocytic leukaemia. British Journal of Haematology. 2007;**139**:762-771

[28] Linet MS, Schubauer-Berigan MK, Weisenburger DD, et al. Chronic lymphocytic leukaemia: An overview of aetiology in light of recent developments in classification and pathogenesis. British Journal of Haematology. 2007;**139**:672-686

[29] Antman KH. The history of arsenic trioxide in cancer therapy. The Oncologist. 2001;**6**(Suppl. 2):1-2

[30] Kwong YL, Tood D. Delicious poison: Arsenic trioxide for the treatment of Leukemia (letter). Blood. 1997;**89**:3487-3488

[31] Gallagher RE. Arsenic -new life for an old poison [editorial]. The New England Journal of Medicine. 1998;**339**:1389-1391

[32] Agency for Toxic Substances and Disease. Registry Arsenic. Retrieved from: http://www.atsdr.cdc.gov/tfacts2.html

[33] Cutler EG, Bradford EH. Action of iron, cod-liver oil, and arsenic on the globular richness of the blood. The American Journal of the Medical Sciences. 1878;**75**:74-84

[34] Forkner CE, Scott TFM. Arsenic as a therapeutic agent in chronic myelogenous leukemia. JAM. 1931;**97**:3-5

[35] Sun HD, Ma L, Hu X-C, et al. Ai-Lin treated 32 cases of acute promyelocytic leukemia. Chinese Journal of Integrated Traditional and Western Medicine. 1992;**12**:170-172

[36] Avvisati G, Mandelli F, Petti MC, Vegna ML, Spadea A, Liso V, et al. Idarubicin (4-demethoxydaunorubicin) as single agent for remission induction of previously untreated acute promyelocytic leukemia: A pilot study of the Italian cooperative group GIMEMA. European Journal of

Haematology. 1990;**44**(4):257-260. DOI: 10.1111/j.1600-0609.1990.tb00389.x

[37] Solis-Herrera A, Ashraf GM, del C A Esparza M, Arias RI, Bachurin SO, Barreto GE, et al. Biological activities of QIAPI 1 as a melanin precursor and its therapeutic effects in Wistar rats exposed to arsenic poisoning. Central Nervous System Agents in Medicinal Chemistry. 2015;**15**:99-108

[38] Ioannidis JPA. Why most published research findings are false. PLoS Medicine. Aug 2005;**2**(8):e124. DOI: 10.1371/journal.pmed.0020124

[39] Lindley DV. A statistical paradox. Biometrika. 1957;**44**:187-192

[40] Starfield B. Is US health really the best in the world? JAMA. 2000;**284**(4):483-486

[41] Weingart SN, Wilson RM, Gibberd RW, Harrison B. Epidemiology and medical error. BMJ. 2000;**320**:774-777